MOLECULAR CARDIOLOGY FOR THE CARDIOLOGIST, SECOND EDITION

MOLECULAR CARDIOLOGY FOR THE CARDIOLOGIST, SECOND EDITION

by

Bernard Swynghedauw, Ph.D., M.D.
Directeur de Recherches à l'INSERM

KLUWER ACADEMIC PUBLISHERS
Boston/Dordrecht/London

Distributors for North, Central and South America:
Kluwer Academic Publishers
101 Philip Drive
Assinippi Park
Norwell, Massachusetts 02061 USA

Distributors for all other countries:
Kluwer Academic Publishers
Distribution Centre
Post Office Box 322
3300 AH Dordrecht, THE NETHERLANDS

Library of Congress Cataloging-in-Publication Data

A C.I.P. Catalogue record for this book is available
from the Library of Congress.

CONTENTS

LIST OF FIGURES.

LIST OF TABLES

PREFACE TO THE SECOND EDITION

For people who are currently doing basic research in medicine the last fifteen years have been quite an exciting period during which new tools available for research appear nearly every week. New biology in 1990 was essentially different from what a 60 year old scientist had learned during his professional education and was based on resynthesizing DNA or RNA fragments and using them for making proteins or detecting rapid, subtle changes in the cardiac or vascular structure.

During the last three years, the progress has been more unbelievable. First, an enormous amount of information concerning differential genetic expression and mutation related to most cardiovascular diseases and risk factors became available and needed to be ranked and linked to physiological functions. Obviously, the reductionist period that we have experienced with molecular biology is going to reach its limits, and more integrative biology needs to be developed, as suggested both by the American Society of Physiology [APS CV Section} and the American Heart Association [Heistad and Fakunding 1997} and during the last meeting of the Federation of European Physiological Societies (FEPS). Second, we now have evidence that within 5 to 7 years we will know the entire structure of human genome and also that of most of the animal species that we currently use in our laboratory. This second explosion in molecular biological science is associated with a radical change in technical approaches. Differential screenings are now becoming rather easily applied and routinely combined with computer research (Internet cloning). Such a reverse biology is opposite to the approach we used during the past ten years and represents a rejection of our experimental designs. Differential screening is indeed like fishing in two different large pools to find different

XX

unknown species of fish, and then trying to identify these species and their role in the ecological organization of the pool. There are indeed no working hypotheses at the beginning except that there are differences in the two pools.

Pathophysiologists will then have the ability to search in a gene bank for the entire sequence of any given mRNA that has been differentially expressed in a diseased tissue and, knowing the gene structure, to deduce the protein sequence and its function (such as, for example, , aldose reductase during the stress response)[Wang and Feuerstein 1997]. Cell biologists have now to determine the role of a number of orphan genes (and proteins) that are detected in the various genetic libraries. Drug companies are now intensively developing such an approach. Physiologists will have at their disposal an incredible number of receptors, which have been identified by analogy by screening a gene library and whose function is unknown (such as, for example, the TIE-2 receptor). Nearly every month, geneticians are identifying new proteins playing important roles in diseased conditions and whose physiological function is unexplored (dystrophin was a good example).

It is now impossible to follow recent progress in cardiology without, at least, knowing the new language that has been created by those practicing new biology because the so-called molecular biology, as every new domain in science, has invented its own mode of expression. This new language does not only include new words that describe new compounds (*intron, exon...*), excessive or needless synonyms (*locus* for place, *segregate* for transmit), but also a new syntax (a gene *encodes* a protein). New words are explained in the glossary at the end of this book.

We have tried to summarize in the most concise way possible the keys that may allow a general practitioner or student who wants to become an internist to read most of the papers published on this matter and to realize where the developments are the most promising from a practical and clinical point of view. There are indeed several important books [Darnel et al. 1986; Kaplan et Delpech 1993; Robert 1993; Marks and Taubman 1997] that introduce the physician to the new biology, but most of them are discouragingly long.

The intent of Molecular Cardiology for the Cardiologist, Second Edition, is to provide a short, easily readable summary of what the new biology brings to cardiology. Special efforts were made to include comprehensive diagrams and drawings, as well as teaching tables, and also to keep the size of the second edition within the modest limits of the first edition. Some of these figures have already been published in various teaching articles [Swynghedauw and Barrieux 1993; Swynghedauw et al. 1993; Swynghedauw et al 1994], and used elsewhere in the course of a rather long career both as a researcher and a teacher in basic cardiology.

The book remains divided into 5 parts. The first part is a general introduction to the new linguistics. This part has been updated by introducing what is sometimes called *Internet biotechnology* and the other various approaches derived from the genome programme. Transgenic technology and gene transfer in autosomal cells are also explained in this chapter and not in the gene transfer chapter as in the previous edition because these techniques are becoming rather routine in most laboratories and publications.

The second part is devoted to the normal structure of the heart and vessels. This area has been covered in relation to the physiological properties of the cardiovascular system, and special care was taken to try to establish bridges between molecular biology and physiology. Several rearrangements were made to facilitate the understanding of receptology, to concentrate ion homeostasis, including pH, into one paragraph, and to better detail the growth processes. The mechanisms of cell death, which were not explained in the previous edition, are now added.

Parts 3 and 4 deal with physiopathology. One of the important contributions of molecular biology to cardiology is a better understanding of the general process of adaptation of the heart and vessels to a permanent mechanical overloading. Such a process is generally called *remodelling,* and results from coordinate changes in the expression of the genes. Thus, heart failure and hypertensive macro angiopathy appear as true diseases of biological adaptation, and it is now possible to provide a biological explanation for most myocardial dysfunction.

Remodelling is essentially different fro the mechanisms that are responsible for genetic disorders. By opposition, genetic diseases result from a modification in the gene structure itself. The study of genetics is rapidly progressing, but its language is particularly hermetic for those who are not familiar with this rather new, or renewed, science. Examples of cardiovascular genetic diseases are given in proportion to the amount of knowledge that we have for each particular disease, which is not, obviously, commensurate with their relative incidence. Nevertheless, more space is devoted to multi genic diseases like arterial hypertension, atherosclerosis, or obesity.

The last part of the book includes information on gene and cellular therapy.

Acknowledgments

This book is dedicated to Pierre-Yves Hatt, a pioneer in molecular cardiology who died a few years ago. He was the first to discover ANF [Marie et al. 1976], and also to show how rapid the changes are in gene expression after the imposition of cardiac overload [Hatt et al, 1965]. I have been working with this outstanding scientist for nearly 15 years, during which time I have learned so much.

I wish to thank my wife, Martine, for her insight and support. I also warmly thank Gérard Delrue, Brigitte Vicens, Annick Allanou, and all their colleagues at INSERM at Le Vésinet for their invaluable contribution to artwork and Gill Butler-Browne for English corrections. I also wish to thank Pascale Benlian (Hopital Saint Antoine, Paris), Daniéle Charlemagne, Claude Delcayre, Christophe Heymes, Jean-Marie Moalic, Lydie Rappaport, Jane-Lyse Samuel (U127-INSERM, Paris), and Bernard Levy (U141-INSERM, Paris) for their critique of my manuscript. The educational and training programme (ETP) committee of the European Society of Cardiology has organized courses on the same topic, and several schemes or ideas presented at this course have been essential to the writing of this edition, especially those from Paul Barton (London), Christian Frelin, and Jacques Barhanin (Nice). Alice Barrieux (Grenoble) gave me precious help in writing the first teaching articles published in *Cardiovascular Research* which were the origin of the present book.

THE NEW LANGUAGE OF BIOLOGY

FROM CHROMOSOME TO GENE.

The first part of this chapter describes the *deoxyribonucleic acid (DNA)* and *ribonucleic acid (RNA)* molecules, their organization within the cell, their synthesis (commonly referred to as *DNA replication* and *RNA transcription* and the regulation of mRNA transcription.

The chemical basis of heredity is shown in Figure 1. 1 which summarizes the concept that every biologist keeps in mind. I resemble my father and also every human being because the biochemical molecules from which I am made are very similar to those from which my parents or other humans are made. In addition, this similarity has been transmitted - geneticians would say *segregated* - during conception. Both the morphology and the main physiological functions of a given human being are expressions of its protein structure. The main physiological functions depend on various enzymes and receptors whose activity is, in turn, a consequence of the spatial structure of a *protein*. Proteins are made from more than 20 amino acids which all have different structures and electric charges. Their final spatial arrangement is entirely determined by these structures and their charges - that is, by the amino acids composition that constitutes the primary structure of the protein.

There are two different levels of spatial arrangement in a protein. The *secondary structure* is the spatial arrangement of the amino acid chain itself - that is its helicity. The *tertiary structure* is formed by the spatial arrangement of the chain which in turn results in the formation of the different pockets where ligands (for the receptors) or substrates (for the

2

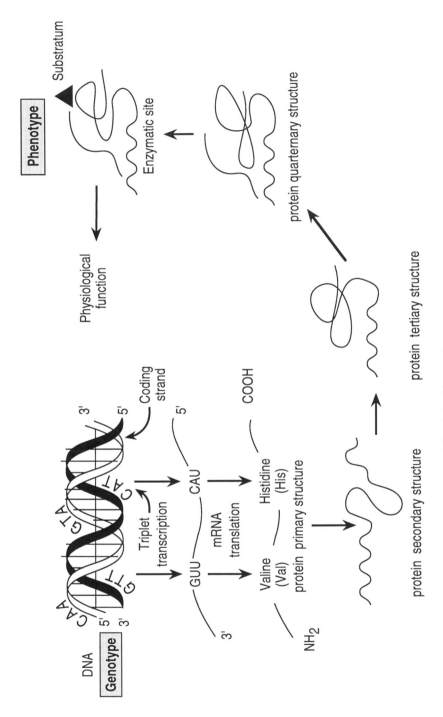

Fig. 1.1. From phenotype to genotype

enzymes) bind. The *quaternary structure* of a protein is the final spatial arrangement of its different subunits, it also reflects the amino acid composition. The amino acid composition is itself determined and transmitted as a *genetic code* provided by a molecule, DNA. Such a dogma is, for the moment, based on a rather limited number of examples. We know the primary structure of most of the proteins and also the composition of nearly all of their corresponding genes. Nevertheless, at the present time the quaternary structure and structure-function relationships has been fully explored for only a few proteins. Such an investigation needs to use several biophysical techniques and also to use transgenic technology and organ physiology in order to establish the correlations between a given part of the molecule and the physiological functions. Strictly speaking the above dogma is in fact a working hypothesis that has never been contradicted.

The *genotype* is the genetic code, and it is present and the same in every nuclei of a given individual. The genotype can be identified in any cell of a given individual, but it can be transmitted to the *progeny* only by the *germinal cells*. The *phenotype* is the apparent manifestation of the genotype, nevertheless phenotype and genotype are different in the same person. For example, the genotype of a cardiac cell and of a hepatocyte are identical in the same individual, but the myocardial phenotype is different from that of the liver, since albumin is present in the liver but not in the heart. It is therefore possible to identify in any cell of an individual an abnormality of the genotype that is responsible for an inherited cardiac disease. There is an intermediary step between the genotype and the phenotype that is taken by RNA, and there is one molecule of special interest, the messenger RNA, *mRNA*, which *transcribes* the genetic code into a language that allows the cellular machine to *translate* the code into a protein.

Chromosome packaging

The genes are the molecules that contain all the information that allows the transcription of an mRNA, but the genes represent a minor portion of the DNA molecule. Most of the molecule is said to be *anonymous* because it is not used to make the phenotype. DNA, proteins responsible for DNA replication and transcription and the first products of the expression of genes are located in highly organized structures present in the cell at *mitosis* and called *chromosomes* (Figure 1. 2). Chromosomes are large structures measured in nmeters, visible by light microscopy, and easily identified by histological techniques in a cell providing the cell is dividing. *Diploid* cells contains an even number of chromosomes - 2 x 23 chromosomes in human - which includes 22 pairs of *autosomal chromosomes*, so-called because they play no role is sex determination, and the 2 sex-determining chromosomes, XX in the female and XY in the male. Diploid cells are called *somatic* cells. The *germinal cells* (or *gametes* and their precursors) are *haploid* and contain only one chromosome from each pair.

Chromosomes can be easily recognized in a chromosomal spread. Each chromosome consists of a pair of *chromatids*. Chromatids are rigorously identical structures that contain exactly the same genetic material and are morphologically identified by having two arms of unequal length. The morphology of chromosomes can be studied using histological techniques that detect distinct bands and enables one to divide the chromosomes into distinct regions. For any animal species, the banding pattern of a given chromosome is reproducible for each staining and is called, for example, Q-banding pattern when the stain is Quinacrine. It allows the identification of the chromosome (chromosome 1, 2, 3,...). Chromosome bands are named by describing the short arm of the chromosome as *p* and the long arm as *q*. Each arm is in turn divided into numbered region, and then further divided into bands and interbands.

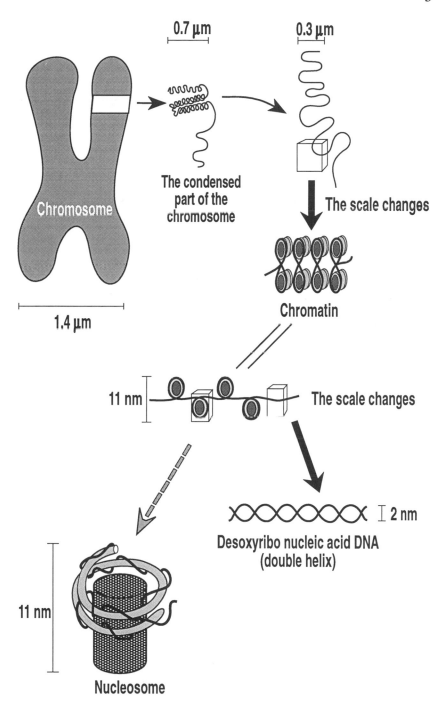

Fig. 1.2. From chromosomes to DNA [from Swynghedauw et al. 1993, with permission from Cardiovasc. Res., 27, 1414]

Chromosomes are located within the cell nuclei. When the cell is not dividing, the chromosomal material is compactly folded into *chromatin* that duplicates before it organizes into chromosomes. After chromatin duplication, the chromosomes containing the same genetic information segregate so that each dividing cell receives exactly the same amount of genetic material. After cell division, the chromosome structure is no longer visible, and the chromatin becomes amorphous.

Chromatin is composed of approximately a one meter-long, 0.2 nanometer-thick string of DNA wound around a core of proteins - *the nucleosomes*. The DNA is also covered with other proteins - structural acidic proteins, transcription factors, and various regulatory factors. The size of each nucleosome is of the order of nmeters. By electron microscopy, nucleosomes appear as beads on a thin string. The beads consist of 2 copies of small basic proteins called *histones*, around which is wound a constant length of DNA and which are separated by DNA bound to a fifth type of histone. Histones are highly conserved between species. The human genome consists of approximately 30 million nucleosomes. Nucleosomes are the cell's mean of packaging a long string of DNA into a very compact structure.

Cell division.

Prokaryotic and *eukaryotic* cells are both able to duplicate their genome and to transmit identical copies of the initial genetic material to daughter cells. Mammalian cells are eukaryotic and divide during their *cell cycle*.

Autosomal cells

Cells from the cardiovascular system are *autosomal cells*. This includes nonmuscular cells such as endothelial cells, fibroblasts, macrophages, and muscle cells such as vascular smooth muscle cells and cardiac myocytes, also called cardiocytes. All these cells divide during development and, at least for the nonmuscular cells, during the adulthood. The division occurs during a cell cycle that is made of several sequential phases: (1) the most variable period is the first gap period, G1, during which the DNA is compactly folded as chromatin and the chromosomes cannot be seen; (2) during the S (S for synthesis) phase (7hours) the double-helical DNA is replicated into two identical daughter DNA molecules, and histones and various proteins responsible for the activity of the chromosome bind rapidly to the new DNA; (3) a second gap period is called G2 (3h), and (4) chromosomes appear as thin threads into the nucleus, and attach to microtubules that have been radiated from the centrioles. Mitosis can then proceed for 1 hour into 4 substages - *prophase, metaphase, anaphase,* and *telophase.* At the end of telophase, *cytokinesis* occurs, and the cell divides into 2 new cells, each of them having the same chromosomes and also chromosomes identical to the chromosomes of the initial cell (Figure 1. 3). Adult cardiocytes do not divide, as neuronal cells (although this dogma has been reconsidered by several authors, and it has been suggested that adult cardiocytes may divide, even in the ventricles, during ischemia) they are quiescent cells which remain in phase G0.

An important issue of the cell cycle of autosomal cells is that the genetic material is copied once. At the beginning, each of the 22 chromosomes exists as a pair, and the cell is 2n. At the end of telophase, immediately before the cell division, each pair of chromosome is doubled and the cell became 4n. After cytokinesis the daughter cells are again 2n and contain exactly the same material as the initial cell - that is a pair of the father's chromosomes and a pair of the mother's chromosome. In addition, there are no crossing-over events in autosomal cells, and the daughter cells are absolutely identical to each other.

8

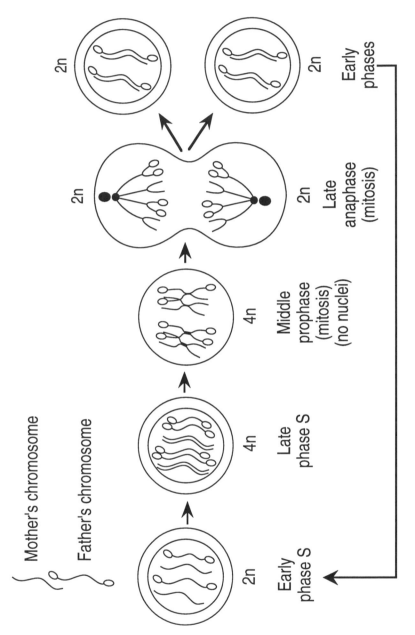

Mother's chromosome

Father's chromosome

2n
Early
phase S

4n
Late
phase S

4n
Middle
prophase
(mitosis)
(no nuclei)

2n

2n
Late
anaphase
(mitosis)

2n

2n

Early
phases

Fig. 1.3.   The cell cycle in autosomal cells: mitosis

Germinal cells

The *germinal cells* have a different cycle, at least at the end of the cycle, and mitosis in these cells is called *meiosis* (Figure 1. 4). During meiosis three important events occur that all contribute to genetic heterogeneity. (1) During the first meiotic division, the chromosomes segregate into the daughter cells randomly with regard to the parental origin. Thus, at least four different types of cells can be generated, as is shown Figure 1. 4. (2) During the first prophase homologous chromosomes align with each other lengthways and make up a sort of ribbon, called *synapsis*, so that each member of the pair consists of homologous chromatids. Subsequently, there are several cuts and ligations that result in an exchange, or *crossing-over,* of genetic material between homologous chromosomes. The point of attachment of the chromatids that participate in the crossing-over is the *chiasma*. This is an important source of genetic variation. In addition, the size of the chromatids segments that have been exchanged determines the *genetic distance* (see Chapter 4). The new chromosomes after the crossing-over are *recombinants.* (3) The third particularity of meiosis is that it includes two divisions: the first results in two cells, which are again 2n; and the second division is different and results into two haploid (1n) cells.

Initially, the pregametic cells contain paired chromosomes, one being from the father, and the other from the mother, and each chromosome is composed by two identical chromatids. Meiosis results in a mixture of genetic information coming from the two parents: we never are identical to our parents, total identity rises only from cloning (an awfull perspective for human beings). The new cells obtained at the end of a meiosis differ from the initial cells, because during the first meiotic division there are both a random mixing of genetic material during the crossing-over and a random distribution of the parental chromosomes. Finally, meiosis involves two separate cell divisions and yields four haploid (1n) cells from one single diploid (2n) cell. Thence we need conception and fusion of one male gamete,

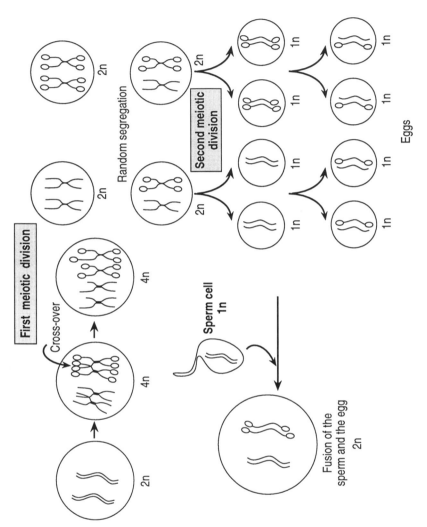

Fig. 1.4. The cell cycle in germinal cells: meiosis

(*spermatozoïde*) and one female gamete (*ovule*), to regenerate a diploid cell, called a zygote, which is an autosomal cell ready for development.

DNA molecule

Biochemistry

The DNA molecule is a dimer composed of a double strand arranged in a helix (the Watson helix) [Watson et al. 1987) (Figure 1. 5). The figure shows 4 turns of the helix and the elementary unit of each strand - the nucleotide (a phosphosugar to which is attached a basic ring). The single strand is a chain of nucleotides linked together by covalent bonds between the phosphate groups and the sugars, the sugar-phosphate backbone. Four different bases are found in each DNA strand - 2 purines adenine, A, and guanine, G, and 2 pyrimidines, cytosine, C, and thymine, T. Each base has a specific affinity for only one other base: G recognizes C, and A recognizes T. The two strands are held together by noncovalent hydrogen bonds between the bases on each strand. Since G forms hydrogen bonds only with C and A only with T, the nucleotide sequence within one strand can be predicted from the other strand, which is its mirror image; the 2 strands are *complementary*.

Nomenclature

The length of a DNA fragment has to be quantified. The unit of length of the DNA molecule is the *nucleotide*. DNA is double-stranded, and the unit is the number of pairs of bases that compose the nucleotides: we say, for example, that we want to clone a DNA fragment of 56 *base pairs* (or 56 *bp*), the number of pairs of nucleotides involved in hydrogen bonding within the fragment. When single-stranded DNA is used, the unit becomes the nucleotide: for example, if the above DNA fragment is dissociated by heat treatment for experimental purpose and becomes single-stranded, its length becomes 56 nucleotides. The human genome contains around 3×10^9 bp.

The DNA strands are oriented and two frequently utilized symbols are *5'* and *3'* which is quite a puzzling convention. Within the DNA chain, two hydroxyl positions on the sugar, 5' and 3', form phosphoester bonds with phosphate (Fig. 1. 5. bottom; see also Figure 1. 8), but at each end of the chain, only one of these 2 positions is free of phosphoric acid, the 5' or the 3'. The building block of DNA is a 5'-linked triphosphonucleotide molecule. Therefore, the 5' phosphoester building blocks, the nucleotide triphosphates, are added to the 3' hydroxyl end of DNA to synthesize a new DNA molecule. The arrow on the DNA strands in the top of Figure 1. 5 indicates the direction of nucleotide addition, from the phosphate-bound 5' to the phosphate-free 3'. Since nucleotides can be added only in one direction, the synthesis of the two strands occurs in opposite directions, and the 5' end of one strand faces the 3' end of the other. Consequently, the two strands are *antiparallel*. When describing genes, it is common to say, for example, that within Chromosome 4, gene A is located in 5' relative to gene B, or upstream of gene B, which conventionally means on Figure 1. 5 that gene A is on the left, in 5' on the *sense* strand.

DNA replication

Replication (Figure 1. 6) occurs during the S phase of the cell cycle. Such a process doubles the genetic information. Duplication is far from being perfect and is also very sensitive to chemical and physical aggressions, which means that duplication is intimately linked to the process of *repair*. DNA replication is routinely mimicked *in vitro* by using a technique called *polymerase chain reaction (PCR)* (see further Current technologies).

Replication begins by a separation of the two DNA strands that have to be copied. This is an energy-consuming process that breaks the hydrogen bonds which bind the two strands together, and is made by a *helicase*. The

A DNA fragment

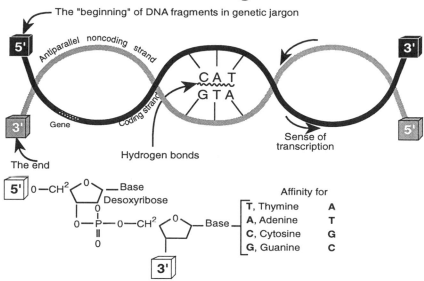

Fig. 1.5. From DNA to nucleotide

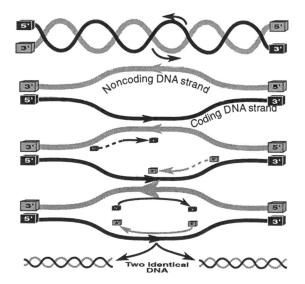

Fig. 1.6. DNA replication
[from Swynghedauw et al., 1993 with permission]

14

process results in the formation of a *replication fork*. The two strands then have to be stabilized by *single strand binding proteins* that form a muff around the two strands. Replication needs to be started by a *primer*, which is a small RNA sequence synthesized by a group of proteins called *primosome* that includes an RNA polymerase. The synthesis of the primer uses the preexisting DNA as a template, is complementary to the DNA sequence to which it binds, and is 3'5' to bind a 5'3' DNA sequence or 5'3' to bind a 3'5' DNA sequence. The synthesis of the whole molecule of DNA is a continuous process on the noncoding strand from 3' to 5'. On the other strand, from 5' to 3', the process is discontinuous and results in several segments called *Okasaki's fragments*. Reparative processes will correct and bind together the Okasaki's fragments. At the end of duplication a specific RNAase will destroy the RNA primers.

Genes and the genetic code

Gene structure

The most important parts of the DNA molecule are the portions of the molecule that contribute to the synthesis of proteins and that are *genes*. A gene includes not only the sequences that code for the protein (the coding DNA), but also a large, and frequently unknown, amount of sequences thatregulate the synthesis of proteins. This means that, in fact, the definition of a given gene is limited by the amount of knowledge that we presently have concerning the regulatory part of this gene. The definition of a gene is indeed more functional than geographical, or physical: this point has considerable consequences. Not all DNA codes for mRNA. The cell needs RNA molecules for other purposes, such as making ribosomes. Even DNA that codes for mRNA contains large segments that never appear in the cytoplasmic mRNA. Finally, most of the DNA never serves for RNA synthesis and is called *silent DNA* or the *anonymous* part of the genome.

A gene is composed of two segments - the regulatory and the coding DNA. In prokaryotes, the coding DNA is unique and uninterrupted. In eukaryotes, the coding DNA is generally (although there are exceptions), located on several fragments of the gene called *exons* (because they are exported to the cytoplasm); the DNA fragments located between the exons are termed *introns* (because they stay inside the nucleus) (Fig. 1. 7). Exons are in the same order as the amino acids in the proteins; nevertheless, as a rule, they do not correspond to a particular functional segment of the protein. Introns were supposed to have no real function, nevertheless this opinion has recently been reevaluated since the discovery that the DNA sequence of introns is, in fact, better organized than that of exons [Peng et al. 1992].

The attachment point of the RNA polymerase is a DNA sequence called the *promotor* which is located upstream of the transcription start site but is not sufficient to permit RNA synthesis. RNA polymerase does not bind directly to DNA but through a group of several proteins. Other DNA sequences that recognize protein factors, the *enhancers*, are also needed.

Genetic code

In the coding DNA, a group of three consecutive nucleotides, the *codon* or *triplet*, corresponds to one amino acid; for example, the triplet CAU corresponds to histidine (Table 1. 1). This is the well-known genetic code. There are 4 nucleotides, A, G, C, and T; therefore there are 4^3 possible codons. There are 64 codons, but since there are only 20 amino acids, some amino acids, the most abundant, are specified by more than one codon.

Starting points and termination points are also specified by specific codons. The initiation triplet encodes for methionine. Stop codons are silentious. The string of nucleotides in the DNA coding strand or in the mRNA determines the final aminoacid sequence in the protein and consequently the final spatial arrangement of the molecule.

16

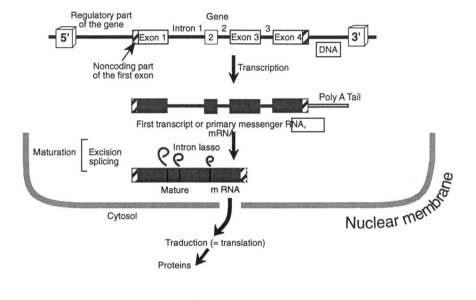

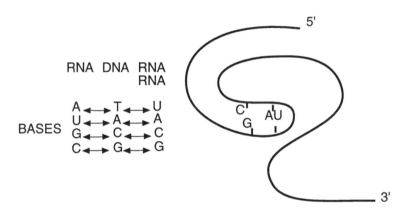

Fig. 1.7. RNA maturation and mRNA structure

Table 1. The genetic code. Bases are in RNA bases, and U is read instead of T. The genetic code is on DNA, and *stricto sensu* it would be preferable to use T, which is on the DNA.

Amino Acids.	Corresponding Triplets.				
Methionine	AUG [start codon]				
Tryptophane	UGG				
Phenylalanine	UUU	UUC			
Histidine	CAU	CAC			
Glutamine	CAA	CAG			
Asparagine	AAU	AAC			
Lysine	AAA	AAG			
Aspartique Acid	GAU	GAC			
Glutamic Acid	GAA	GAG			
Cysteine	UGU	UGC			
Tyrosine	UAU	UAC			
Isoleucine	AUU	AUC	AUA		
Valine	GUU	GUA	GUC	GUG	
Proline	CCU	CCA	CCC	CCG	
Threonine	ACU	ACA	ACC	ACG	
Alanine	GCU	GCA	GCC	GCG	
Glycine	GGU	GGA	GGC	GGG	
Serine	UCU	UCA	UCC	UCG	AGU	AGC
Leucine	CUU	CUA	CUC	CUG	UUA	UUG
Arginine	CGU	CGA	CGC	CGG	AGA	AGG
[Codons stops]	UAA	UAG	UGA		

Because the arrangement of the bases specifies the aminoacid arrangement, the sequence of the bases in the coding DNA strand is identical to the mRNA and codes for the aminoacid sequence, the coding DNA sequence being read from the 5' to the 3' direction; 5' specifies for the amino end of the protein and 3' for its carboxyl end (Figure 1. 8). The other strand of DNA, which is the mirror image of the coding strand is the noncoding or antisense DNA strand. The RNA polymerase attaches at the 3' end of the non-coding strand of DNA, the antisense strand. It brings in and links together the nucleotides complementary to the strand to which it is attached - for example a C when G is on the DNA, an A when T is on the DNA. The new RNA molecule is transcribed from the noncoding antisense DNA strand but only complementary to this strand. It is identical to the coding DNA strand. In Figure 1. 8, the RNA polymerase has finished to transcribe and is consequently located on the 5' end of the non coding DNA strand.

In molecular biology, *parallel* or *antiparallel* either are verbs or qualify a strand relative to another: mRNA parallels the coding DNA strand, the two DNA strands are antiparallel. DNA strands are named using several synonyms: the coding strand is also called 5'-3', sense strand, or antiparallel (to the other).

Main types of genes

During evolution meiotic division has frequently resulted in the multiplication of identical copies of a given gene, sometimes with a few differences that do not modify gene function but also sometimes with major modifications that suppress the coding function of the gene and results in *pseudogenes*. The actin gene, for example, exists as 50 to 70 copies with identical, or similar sequences or pseudogenes. The degree of *homology* of two sequences indicates the percentage of nucleotides that are exactly at the

19

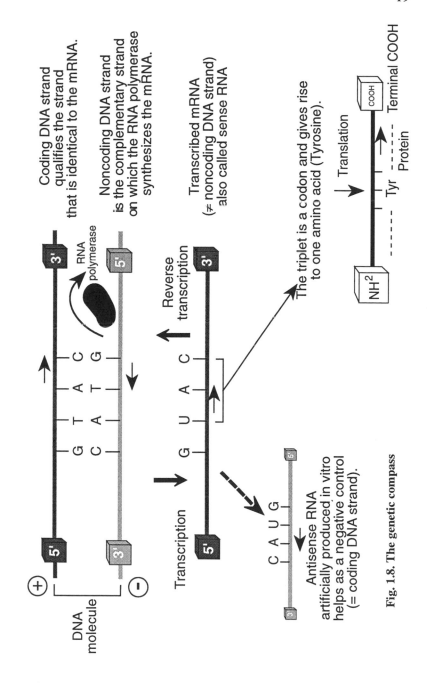

Coding DNA strand qualifies the strand that is identical to the mRNA.

Noncoding DNA strand is the complementary strand on which the RNA polymerase synthesizes the mRNA.

Transcribed mRNA (≠ noncoding DNA strand) also called sense RNA

The triplet is a codon and gives rise to one amino acid (Tyrosine).

Antisense RNA artificially produced in vitro helps as a negative control (= coding DNA strand).

Fig. 1.8. The genetic compass

same place on the two sequences. Nucleotide sequences are said to be highly homologous when the degree of homology is between 75 to 100%.

In mammals, most of the genes are composed by exons of different length, which are separated from each other by introns, which also may have extremely different lengths. The number of exons is variable from one gene to another: the human gene coding for the myosin heavy chain (MHC) isoform β (molecular weight, MW: 200,000) has 43 exons; by contrast, the gene of the fast isoform of Troponin I (TNI) has only 8 exons. These two proteins are also good examples to show that exons and functional sites are not superimposable: on the β MHC the actin binding site is spread over 2 full exons (14 and 15) and a portion of two others (13 and 16); on TNI the binding site for Troponin C is spread over two exons (4 and 5); whereas the actin binding site on the same molecule is entirely located on exon 7. Another important point is that genes from different animal species and encoding the same molecule may have a completely different structure. For example, the gene encoding myosin heavy chain in Drosophilea 36B is composed of 19 exons instead of 40 in humans. There are also intronless genes, which are supposed to be genes of bacterial origin that have been incorporated into the mammalian genome during evolution and maintained as such because of an evolutionary advantage. This group of genes includes histones and the genes encoding the adrenergic and muscarinic receptors.

It is now common to try to rearrange genes into families or superfamilies, based on both genetic structure and functional phenotype. A good example are the genes coding for nuclear hormonal receptors - that is progesterone, oestrogenes, gluco- and mineralocorticoides, and thyroxine receptors that have in common a specific N terminal sequence, DNA binding, and ligand binding domains, and, of course, the fact that they are hormonal receptors. The so-called R7G receptor family includes the adrenergic and muscarinic genes receptors as well as the receptors for angiotensin II. These genes are usually intronless and possess 7 transmembrane hydrophobic domains and a G protein subunit binding site. They encode hormonal membrane receptors (see Chapter 2). Such a *taxonomy* is currently going to be entirely reconsidered based on findings from The Human Genome Sequencing Program (see below).

Isogenes.

Genes and proteins are not superimposable notions, and moreover there are genes that can encode several proteins. *Isoforms* are different proteins with the same function; *isoenzymes* are enzymes with the same function and slight differences in their activity and structure. Nevertheless, the genes coding for a group of isoforms can be unique or multiple. Multigenic families include different genes, called *isogenes*, sometimes located in different chromosomes, coding for isoforms or isoenzymes.

In cardiovascular research a good example of this is the genes coding for the cardiac myosin heavy chain isoforms α and β. These genes are distinct and reflect differences both in the amino acid composition of the protein and the enzymatic activity. They are located on the same chromosome in an antithetic manner. The skeletal muscle embryonic, neonatal and fast isoforms are also coded by a series of genes located on a different chromosome. By contrast, there are genes such as those that encode for tropomyosin that are able to code for several different isoforms by the process of alternative *splicing*. In this case, one exon of the gene is common to all isoforms, and alternative splicing allows the gene to express only one or several exons specific for the given isoform.

The human genome sequencing program

Several bacterial genomes have already been fully sequenced so far (Table 1. 2), nevertheless, the size of mammalian genomes creates per se specific problems that are yet not fully resolved. Human or mouse genomes are 3,000-fold the size of that of most of bacteria, and only 60 million base

22

pairs out of 3 billion have been analyzed to date [Rowen et al. 1997]. The expressed genes are rather easily analyzed from cDNA libraries, and approximately half of the 100,000 human genes sequences are present in a public database to date.

Table 1. 2. Current status of genomic sequences in 1997 (from Rowen et al. 1997)

Organism	Genome size, Mb	Percentage sequenced
11 microbacteria	0.6 to 4.2	100
Escherichia coli	4.6	100
Yeast	13	100
Nematode	100	70
Drosophila	130	6
Mouse	3,000	0.2
Human	3,000	2

The Human Genome Project, which is now a huge industry, is developed around few *sequencing centers* and an increasing number of new technologies (for example, for identifying continuous arrays of sequence-ready clones and the corresponding overlapping zones, also termed *tiling paths*), including a new discipline, *bioinformatics*. There are periodically up-dated reports on the state of the project. The program includes multiple libraries, and because the rate of polymorphism in human is about one variation per 500 bp, including insertions and deletions, there are differences in the available fingerprints. The program is also based on *genetic markers* (like microsatellites), whose number is growing every month. Such markers allow geographical identifications on the whole genome [Weissenbach

1996]. Another major strategical problem to be resolved is that, from a pure technical point of view, it is preferable to use a minimum number of highly redundant clone libraries, while social and ethical considerations will argue for deverse clone libraries [Rowen et al. 1997]. The genome project might be completed by 2005, provided that improvements in biotechnology continue at the same speed that they now are occurring [Weissenbach 1996].

Gene classification

A universal gene classification system is now a quite urgent need. The challenge is to organize the enormous complexity of data provided by the genome programs. In contrast with the Linnaeus classification, which was based on the phenotype of the various members of the evolutional tree, the actual *taxonomy* is based on genotype. Comparisons between different complete genome sequences allowed the delineation of protein families based on sequence similarities. Several levels of organization have then been delineated [Tatusov et al. 1997, Henikoff et al. 1997]. (1) *Orthologs* genes are genes from different species that evolve from a common ancestral gene by speciation and retain the same function in the course of evolution. Typically, ortholog genes form a collection of genes sharing the same ancestry and performing the same role in different organisms. The first approach would be to accept that ortholog genes are genes from two different genomes with the highest sequence similarity. Identification of these orthologs is then critical for predicting new gene function and interpreting phylogenetic trees. (2) *Paralog* genes are genes that are related by duplication within a genome and that evolve new functions, such as, for example, α- and β-globins and myoglobin that arose from duplications of ancestral globin genes but have different functions. (3) In fact, at large phylogenetic distances, the situation is much more complicated. A first approach, based on known bacterial, mycoplasma, and archaeal proteins, was proposed by Tatusov et al. [1997]. All pairwise sequences comparisons among the genes from seven genomes that have been entirely sequenced were performed, and for each of these genes the best hit in each of other genomes was calculated and detected. Then, sequence similarities allowed to delineate 720 *clusters of orthologous groups (COG)* in genomes from five different phylogenetic lineages. Such COGs contain both individual orthologous genes and orthologous sets of paralogs that are descendants of a single ancestral gene and correspond to an ancient conserved region. COGs are associated with a conserved specific function (such as transcription, lipid metabolism, amino acid metabolism, and tranport). Such a taxonomic approach allow to delineate phylogenetic patterns that are specific for given lineages.

Structural inferences made from DNA sequences alignments are valuable for searching new proteins and new functions, and orthologous and paralogous relationships are now the genomic basis of protein families and superfamilies. The smallest conserved sequence of a given protein family is termed *motif*. *Modules* (also called *domains* or *building blocks*) are contiguous sequence segments that can consist of a single or multiple motifs in fixed order. The resulting protein can be made from a single module or concatenation of several modules, and gene familie can be tndemly duplicated or dispers throughout the genome [Henikoff et al. 1997]. Some modules are present throughout the whole evolution tree (such as the ATP-binding cassette), while others appear at a given moment of the evolution (such as the homeodomain or the C2H2 Zn finger). Good examples were given below in the Chapter 2 in the Ion channels and electrical activity section. The structure of the voltage-gated ion channels principal subunit was composed by the same module that surrounds the central pore and consists in six transmembrane hydrophobic helices that are easily detectable in a gene bank and are motifs. The detection of a particular motif in a sequence data bank is a good strategy for detecting new functions; nevertheless there are many proteins that contain several modules from a variety of different families (see below the tyrosine kinase receptors on

Figure 2. 25) and multiple solutions for the same critical cellular function appear to be the rule rather than an exception, at least in phylogeny. Several mechanisms, including homologous recombination, inversions, duplications and translocations contributed to the dispersion of these protein building blocks, and chasing functionnaly significant motifs or modules or duplicated products of motifs through the Internet is one of the favorite games of contemporary biologists.

Transcription

Transcription occurs on the noncoding strand of DNA and is the synthesis of an RNA molecule that is identical to the coding strand of DNA. Transcription is just a copy. Reverse transcription is also a copy, and occurs *in vivo,* in cells infested with retrovirus. It is also a useful research tool, since it allows one to synthesize routinely in the test tube DNA, called complementary DNA (*cDNA*) from mRNA (Figure 1. 8). Reverse transcription is routinely used because DNA is less fragile than RNA and cDNA is easier to handle than RNA or cRNA.

Transcription is a complex process and involves numerous steps : (1) binding of RNA polymerases to the DNA and recognition of relevant sequences; (2) opening of the double-stranded DNA; (3) binding of the substrates (that is the ribonucleotides); (4) initiation, which consists of the formation of the first two phosphodiester bonds; (5) elongation (both initiation and elongation also exist during translation into proteins) by further polymerization with ribonucleotides and movement along the DNA template, which is the noncoding strand of the double helix and (6) release of the RNA chain. The activity of the RNA polymerases themselves depends on a group of transcription factors that are proteins. Polymerases and transcription factors unwind the DNA molecule, maintain the transcription bubble constant during the making of RNA, and separate the new nascent RNA molecule from the DNA.

26

Biotechnology allows to produce in vitro the mirror image of the mRNA, the *complementary RNA (cRNA)* (Figure 1. 8), also called the *antisense RNA* which is identical to the antisense DNA strand. The antisense RNA gene is a tool that has many uses, including transgenic technology and gene therapy.

The RNA molecule

Structure

The cell synthesizes three different types of RNA: *messenger RNA (mRNA)* which translates the genetic code into proteins and is the least abundant; *ribosomal RNA (rRNA)* which is the most abundant, and *transfer RNA (tRNA)* which is the RNA that transports the amino acids to the site of the translation. A specific RNA polymerase corresponds to each of different types of RNA (RNA polymerase I for rRNA, II for mRNA, and III for tRNA). RNAs are synthesized in a 5' to 3' direction from one strand of DNA called *template DNA*. RNA and its DNA template are antiparallel and have complementary nucleotides, but RNA and the DNA strand complementary to the template are parallel (Figures 1. 5 and 1. 8). In other words, RNA has the same 5' to 3' orientation and the same nucleotide sequence as the 5'-3' antisense DNA strand (with one exception, T does not exist in RNA and is replaced by U).

Figure 1. 7 shows schematically the structure of a mRNA molecule. The sequence of nucleotides present in the transcribed RNA is almost identical to the DNA coding strand: U in the RNA molecule forms hydrogen bonds with A, and A with T, G with C, and C with G. Naturally occurring RNA is a single strand. But if, within the single strand, there are strings of bases that are complementary, the single-stranded RNA will loop on itself to form shortlength double stranded-stems. These stems have important physiological consequences for the different RNA species present in the cell and may also represent a difficult problem when mRNA is manipulated because the RNA strand can hybridize to itself.

Synthesis

Figure 1. 7 shows the different steps involved in synthesis and maturation of mRNA. The coding strand of a gene is composed of exons and introns. Introns are transcribed, but they are not coding; however not all exons are coding. A portion of the first and last exons is noncoding, and their ends are modified. The 5' end of the first exon is blocked by a 5' to 5' sugar-phosphate covalent bond called the *RNA cap*. To the last exon is attached a string of repetitive A, AAAAA..., called the *poly(A) tail*; hence the other name of mRNA, is poly(A)-rich RNA. This property is used both to quantify and isolate the total mRNAs. The poly(A) tail is thought to increase the efficiency at which mRNA is translated into proteins; the mRNA cap is necessary for the initiation of protein synthesis.

Introns are transcribed into premRNA, also called *nuclear mRNA*. They need to be eliminated by excision. In order to be excised, the introns form loops called *lariats* that are degraded in the nucleus. The exons are then joined together by ligation. The two process of excision and ligation are called *splicing*. Transcription, splicing, and attachment of the poly(A) tail represent the different steps of the mRNA maturation and constitute an important step of regulation control. mRNA is finally transported to the cytoplasm to be translated into protein on the ribosomal machinery via aminoacyl tRNAs.

Regulation of gene expression

Gene expression is regulated at the level of the regulatory part of the gene located upstream of the coding sequence of a gene (in 5') [Wingender 1993]. This DNA segment is of variable length, and the nucleotides are negatively

28

named from the start codon: - 240 bp means that we are located 240 bp upstream from the start codon. The regulatory part of the gene includes two different segments: one is usually close to the first exon and is called the *promotor*, and the other which is called the *enhancer* and is upstream of the promotor. The spatial configuration of the gene is such that the enhancer can be close to the promotor and have structural connections with it.

In Figure 1. 9, two DNA consensus sequences are shown in the promotor region - the TATA box and the CAAT box that binds RNA polymerase through specific proteins. Both contain a consensus DNA sequence with invariant and variable nucleotides. The enhancers also have consensus sequences that are different and bind specific transcriptional factors: glucocorticoid responsive element (GRE) that binds glucocorticoid receptors, cAMP responsive element (CRE) or triiodothyronine responsive element (TRE) and so on.

The regulation of gene transcription proceeds in two steps: the first step is a *transregulation* and consists of the synthesis of a transcriptional factor, usually on a different chromosome but at the least by genes different from the regulated gene. Transregulation occurs when the transcriptional factor binds to the enhancer. Transregulation is the result of a protein/DNA interaction. Cis-regulation occurs on DNA, when the regulator is contiguous to the gene (Figure 1. 10). Enhancers and the promotor are cis-regulators.

Figure 1. 11 summarizes what we know about the hormone regulation of gene expression. There are two main classes of hormone receptors: transmembrane and nuclear receptors. When hormones such as isoproterenol or insulin bind to their transmembrane receptors, they generate a signal that is transduced into a second intracellular signal. The signal is cAMP for isoproterenol which binds protein kinase A; this, in turn, phosphorylates a transcriptional factor that binds DNA at the level of the cAMP responsive element. The signal is the activation of a cascade of

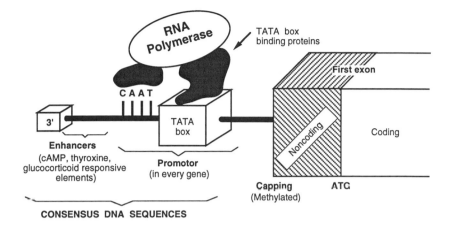

Fig. 1.9. The regulatory part of a gene

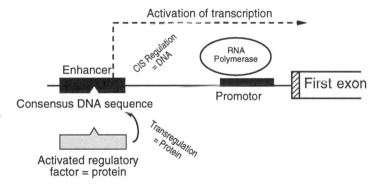

The factor can be activated by a hormone, by phosphorylation, by cAMP, by dimerization, or by dissociation from an inhibitory protein.

Fig. 1.10. Cis and transregulation [from Swynghedauw and Barrieux 1993 with permission from Cardiovasc. Res., 27, 1414]

30

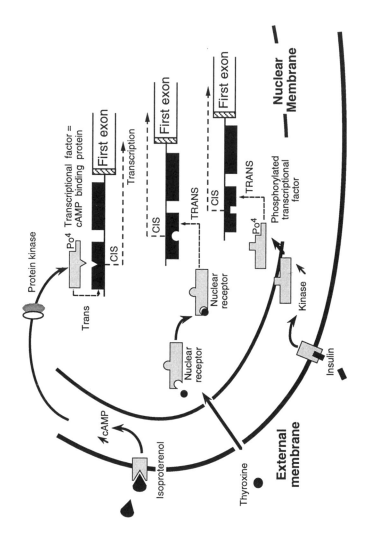

Fig. 1.11. Transcriptional regulation of hormone effects
[from Swynghedauw and Barrieux 1993, with permission from Cardiovasc. Res., 27, 1414]

kinases for insulin. The net result in both examples is the phosphorylation of enhancer binding proteins by specific kinases. These phosphorylated transacting factors bound to their respective responsible element activate the RNA polymerase already attached to the promotor. In either case, the hormone transported into the cytoplasm forms a complex with its specific receptor, and the complex bound to its responsive element in the nucleus once again activates the promotor-bound polymerase.

The receptors that belong to the nuclear hormonal receptors family bind to hydrophilic hormones such as thyroxine or aldosterone and are directly activated by the hormone. Activated receptors can bind the corresponding DNA consensus sequence without any intermediary proteins. It is important to note that the knowledge of the existence of a given consensus sequence - lets say a glucose-responsible element - in the regulatory portion of a gene is not sufficient to attribute such a type of regulation to the gene expression; it needs physiological investigations in order to have the true demonstration of this type of activation.

CURRENT TECHNOLOGIES

Molecular biology offers a broad range of techniques that are largely responsible for several misunderstandings occurring during the cross-talk between clinicians. The reader may refer to several excellent laboratory manuals to find technical details related to this chapter [Sambrook et al. 1989; Kriegler 1990].

Basic tools: probes, stringency, and restriction enzymes

Probes (Figure 1. 12) in molecular biology are nucleotide sequences, radioactively or non radioactively labeled, which are used for identification, mostly after specific hybridation with a complementary nucleotide sequence

32

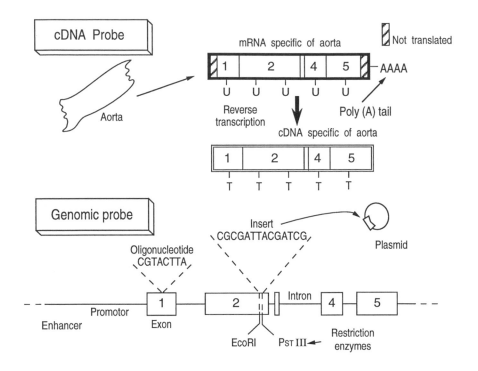

Fig. 1.12. Genetic probes

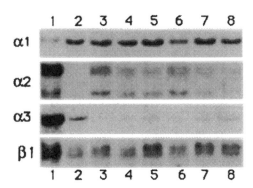

Fig. 1.13. Northern blot analysis: Na, K-ATPase α isoforms and β1 subunit mRNAs in rat tissues.
1-neonatal brain; 2-neonatal heart ; 3 and 6-normal adult heart; 4 and 7-cardiac hypertrophy (between 40 and 50 %); 5 and 8-cardiac hypertrophy (between 60 and 90 %) [from Charlemagne et al. 1994 with permission].

(Figure 1. 13). The most commonly used probes are cDNA probes, genomic probes and oligonucleotides. (1) cDNA represents only that part of DNA that is transcribed in a specific tissue. cDNA originates from reverse transcription of mature mRNAs. Mature mRNAs vary from one tissue to another during development or in disease states. cDNA is a copy of the exons that are mostly coding but also contains, at the beginning of the first exon and at the end of the last one, a noncoding sequence (Figure 1. 8). (2) In contrast, genomic DNA is isolated directly from the DNA of nuclei and is the same in every cell of an individual. The genomic DNA of a gene contains exons, introns, and the regulatory part of the gene located upstream the first exon. It contains all the hereditary information that makes this individual unique. (3) *Oligonucleotides* have been commercially synthesized. Their length is around 20 to 40 nucleotides Usually they are complementary to a small portion of mRNA or DNA. The most commonly utilized primers are oligonucleotides. There are now several techniques to synthesize radioactive cDNA probes. Commercial kits are available for all of them.

A large part of biotechnologies consists of making DNA-DNA or DNA-RNA hybrids. The unknown DNA or RNA sequence is subsequently identified thanks to the radioactive DNA (or sometimes RNA) probe. The two hybrids are bound by a hydrogen bond that is stable in given conditions of temperature and ionic strength. For example, the two DNA strands can be separated by heating, and this is a well-known tool for preparing single-stranded DNA. The two DNA strands are fully separated at a given temperature, and the intermediary temperature (called *Tm*) is a reproducible physical characteristic of a given DNA molecule. The lower the ionic strength, the lower the *Tm*. *Stringency* is the product of temperature and ionic strength, and a solution with high stringency is a solution with a low ionic strength and/or high temperature. Every probe hybridizes to its complementary sequences in given stringency conditions, and the determination of the most appropriate conditions of stringency is the first step to allow the quantification of a nucleotide sequence.

Restriction enzymes are the main enzymes used in molecular biology: they are endonucleases that were discovered in bacteria by a Noble prize winner and have the property of cleaving sequences present in the double-stranded DNA (Figure 1. 14). Both strands are cut - sometimes in a staggered manner to give "sticky ends", sometimes at the same nucleotide on both strands to give "blunt ends" as for Alu I. Most of the restriction enzymes cleaves *palindromic* sequences on the two DNA strands at a very specific site in terms of nucleotides; nevertheless there are also restriction enzymes capable of cleaving sequences that are only partially defined, such as Nsp II. The DNA sequences wthat can be cleaved by a restriction enzyme are called *restriction sites*. There are several hundreds of these enzymes, and their nomenclature is based on the bacteria from which the enzyme has been isolated; for example, Eco R1 was isolated from the RY13 strain of Escherichia coli. Most of the restriction enzymes are specific for a given sequence, so they are tools for identifying DNA sequences and for providing a rapid idea of the nucleotide sequence. Figure 1. 14 shows the conventional representation of a nucleotide sequence, such as a gene that is seen in every article describing a new gene. It includes a scale in base pairs, the length and position of both exons (always represented as boxes) and introns (represented as thin lines), and the position of the restriction sites. Obviously, the more numerous the sites the more precise the definition, and it has empirically been shown that a gene sequence can be identified with enough accuracy when 2 to 3 restriction sites are indicated.

Restriction maps (Figure 1. 15) result from the electrophoresis of the fragments obtained after digesting of a given DNA sequence with restriction enzymes. Following digestion, the fragments are separated by electrophoresis according to their molecular weights and can be identified using BET for example, a fluorescent (and toxic) chemical that binds every

A. Restriction enzyme

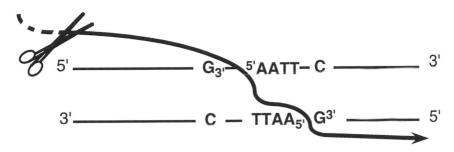

Cut palindromic sequences on the two DNA strands
Eco R1 = First restriction, enzyme found in Echerichia Coll Ry13

B. Restriction sites

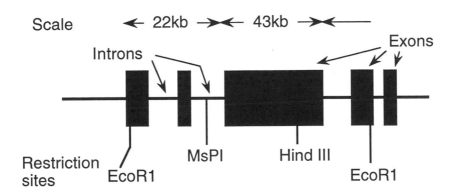

Conventional representation of a gene

Fig. 1.14. Restriction enzymes (A) and restriction site (B)
[from Swynghedauw et al. with permission from Cardiovasc. Res, 21, 1566]

36

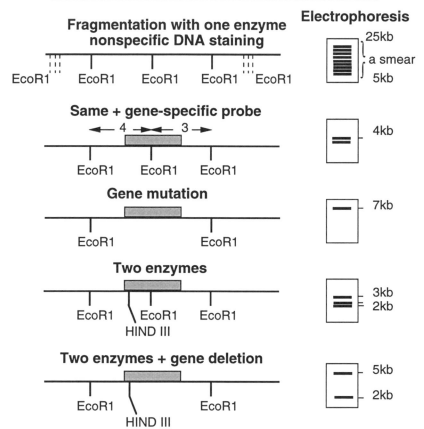

Fig. 1.15. Restriction maps [from Swynghedauw et al. 1993, with permission from Cardiovasc. Res., 27, 1566]

DNA fragment may show a broad smear if applied, for example, to a complex mixture of genomic DNA and is then useless. To obtain a real map, we need a second component, which is usually a radioactive single-stranded probe, specific for a given region of the DNA molecule - for example, a known, well-identified, portion of a gene. Then the probe allows a geographical localization of the DNA fragments, by specific hybridization to a given fragment which has previously been separated by electrophoresis. It then becomes possible to analyze the fragments generated by the restriction enzymes and obtain a sort of fingerprint of the gene. Historically, restriction mapping was a very effective way to identify (and understand) DNA polymorphism.

Polymerase Chain Reaction (PCR).

This technique is based on the principle of DNA duplication (Figure 1. 6). As stated previously, DNA replication needs a complete dissociation of the two DNA strands as a prerequisite and also the synthesis of two primers that hybridize specifically to a given segment of the two strands and limit the portion of DNA to be duplicated. *In vivo* there are enzymes that denature the DNA and synthesize the primers. Once a primer is provided, DNA polymerase may synthesize a coding DNA strand by using the DNA noncoding strand as a guideline and vice-versa. The result is two identical molecules of DNA.

It is possible to reproduce this process *in vitro* by using heat to dissociate the two DNA strands and by synthesizing oligonucleotides (around 20 nucleotide length) to make primers complementary to the two extremities of the DNA sequence of interest [Becker-André and Hahlbrock 1989; Wang et al. 1989]. It is therefore possible to repeat such a duplication process nearly indefinitely until we have amplified the sequence in such quantities that we can see the newly made DNA by electrophoresis. We have to add to the mixture the appropriate nucleotides and DNA polymerase. Nevertheless the repetition of such an amplification needs several cycles of heating that destroys the DNA polymerase, and the amplification procedure was impossible until the discovery of Thermophilus aquaticus (*Taq*) and its heat-resistant DNA polymerase. The PCR can usually repeat the operation 20 to 30 times and then amplify a DNA strand 100, 1,000 and even 10^6 times.

PCR is performed in a small inexpensive apparatus and can be programed to produce cycles of temperature that can be repeated numerous times: 95°C dissociates the two DNA strands, 55°C allows the primers to hybridize to each DNA strand, 72°C allows the polymerase to synthesize DNA, then begin again of the cycle (Figure 1. 16).

When mRNA is to be amplified, it has to be transformed into a single-stranded DNA by using reverse transcriptase (Figure 1. 8). The primers are either 5'-3' and will anneal to the 3' end of the non-coding strand, or 3'-5'. Only the portion of the sequence that is contained between the two primers will be amplified. During the first cycle, the synthesis of the DNA strands is not limited in length and will go as far as the polymerase chooses to go on the DNA template (Figure 1. 16). However, in subsequent cycles, the length of the new strands is limited to the region of DNA recognized by the primers, since after the first cycle strands will stop where the primer has started in the previous cycle.

The amplification procedure produces a large amount of a single DNA fragment that can be quantified on a gel. One of the problems in obtaining quantitative results is that the number of amplification cycles is always unknown, mainly because some cycles remain unfinished. Therefore, it is necessary to coamplify an internal probe to really obtain quantitative results. Two groups of probes can be utilized. The most commonly utilized is an already present transcript that is supposed not to be modified by the experimental procedure that we are going to perform. Glucose-6-phosphate

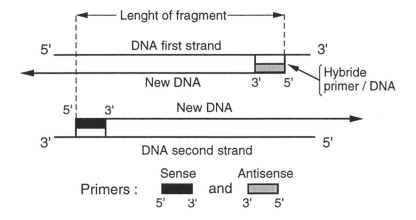

Primers :   Sense   and   Antisense

The first cycle gives rise to fragments that are too long.

DNA polymerase
3 different temperatures

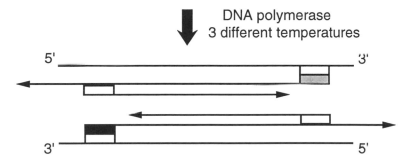

The other cycles give fragments of limited length.

n cycles

Amplification (~ 15 to 30)

Fig. 1.16. Polymerase chain reaction (PCR) [from Swynghedauw et al. 1993, with permission from Cardiovasc. Res., 27, 1566]

dehydrogenase or actin are commonly used in cardiovascular research: nevertheless, they have to be utilised with cautious because both can change - for example during the process of hypertrophy. It is now preferable to use a sense RNA very alike the mRNA of interest to avoid formation of hybrids. This could be obtained *in vitro* by transcribing the sequence of interest previously inserted into a special plasmid that contains two different promoters, one on each side of the cDNA insert. It thus permits the transcription of both antisense RNA (which is a negative control) and sense RNA (see Figure 1. 8). Then the molecular weight of the new *transcript* has to be slightly modified to render the probe detectable on electrophoresis, which is usually performed by introducing into the RNA sequence either a deletion or a small insert. The results are expressed as a ratio between the standart and the mRNA of interest.

This technique is now a major tool for routine molecular biology. It is at the origin of many of the major recent progresses that have been made in genetics and also is the basis of the *serial analysis of gene expression (SAGE)* (see below). It has many applications, including mRNA quantification, even on histological slices, detection of repetitive DNA sequences, synthesis of various DNA fragments in detectable quantities, and so on. PCR has been extensively applied in cardiovascular research, and numerous examples are given on nearly every page below. It is now possible to extract total RNA from 3 to 5 mg samples of human heart and to reverse transcribe this RNA into cDNA [Feldman et al. 1991].

Working with RNA

Quantifying mRNA in cardiology
Obviously mRNAs are not protein. They don't possess any functional activity except making proteins. Nevertheless, their quantification provides

information of crucial importance both in cardiovascular physiology and pharmacology.

(1) The techniques used to quantitate mRNAs, including slot blot analysis and quantitative PCR, are often easy and rapid, and it is possible to quantify several messengers at the same time. This has to be compared with the classical biochemistry, which is time consuming. A good example comes from studies on the Na^+, K^+ ATPase, the sodium pump that maintains cell depolarization and binds ouabain. During mechanical overload of the heart, the expression of the gene coding for the a subunit of this enzyme is modified, resulting in modifications of the enzymatic activity and pharmacological properties. To demonstrate that the enzymatic function and sensitivity to ouabain were changed required 4 years [Lelièvre et al. 1986], while the molecular biological results were completed within 6 months [Charlemagne et al. 1994] (Figure 1. 13).

(2) During physiological steady states, such as senescence [Besse et al. 1993] or after chronic administration of a drug, such as a converting enzyme inhibitor, mRNA levels generally correlate with the corresponding protein concentration, so that RNA quantitation may be equated with protein content. However, one should be aware that such a relationship is far from being the rule. There are a lot of exceptions - for example collagen, which is certainly not fully transcriptionnally regulated in the heart [Besse et al. 1993].

(3) Rapid biological transitions, such as those obtained after acute mechanical overload [Bauters et al. 1988; Delcayre et al. 1992], hormonal injection, or acute administration of a drug, represent a major concern in cardiology. mRNA levels may be altered long before there is any detectable change in the corresponding proteins. Nevertheless, it is also important to know that transcripts may change without any translation into proteins [Snoeckx et al. 1991].

(4) The routine strategy to identify the level of regulation of a given modification in protein level (Figure 1. 7), includes the determination of the corresponding mRNA level. Nevertheless it is important to know that, by so doing, we are not measuring transcription. An increased mRNA level is frequently the result of increased gene transcription, but it may also result from modifications occurring at any steps of mRNA maturation in the nucleus. For example, during chronic cardiac overload in rats a shift occurs in the different myosin isoforms [Lompré et al. 1979]. It has been shown that this shift is preceded by a change in the corresponding mRNAs. The change in mRNAs occurs roughly 2 to 3 days before that of the proteins [Lompré et al. 1979] which allows one to conclude that the regulation is pretranslational and that the chicken is the mRNA and the egg is the protein. By contrast, during aging, the myocardial collagen mRNA concentration decreases while the protein content increases [Besse et al. 1994].

The role of transcription can be determined only by using other techniques. Transcriptional run-on is one of them and consists of studying transcription directly on isolated nuclei. It allows one to know if the increased mRNA level is also accompanied by a parallel augmentation of premRNAs (those that contain transcribed introns, Figure 1. 7). By so doing, it has, for example, been demonstrated that the cardiac myosin level is mainly regulated at the transcriptional level [Boheler et al. 1992]. Another possibility is to use transgenic technology or transfection.

How to prepare and handle RNA

A major problem in working with RNA is RNase contamination. Most RNases are heat-stable and are present everywhere including on the fingers of investigators. In the cardiovascular system, RNAases start to destroy tissue RNA soon after death which renders postmortem tissue determination of mRNA impossible. This is the reason that biopsy samples taken during open-heart surgery, transplantation, or catheterism have to be rapidly stored in liquid nitrogen. Nevertheless, working on RNA is possible in nearly any cardiovascular laboratory providing a minimum of care (such as disposable gloves, heat-baked glassware and so on) is taken.

mRNA needs to be quantified total RNA that is protein- and DNA-free. This is done on fresh or deep-frozen tissues. One of the most popular techniques in our domain is based on rapid homogenization in a chaotropic agent to inactivate RNases, followed by an extraction in acidic phenol/chloroform to remove proteins and DNA, precipitation of the RNA by alcohol, solubilization of the remaining double-stranded nucleic acids but not single-stranded ribosomal, and mRNA in high salt solutions and several cycles of solubilization-reprecipitation in ethanol [Chomczynski and Sacchi 1987]

It may be necessary to isolate pure mRNAs for various purposes. The isolation procedure is usually based on the principle of affinity chromatography and exploits a structural property specific to mRNAs that is a poly(A) tail at the 3' end of mRNA (Figure 1. 7). Such a tail can hybridize to complementary bases, uridine or thymidine, in high ionic strength, and dehybridize at low ionic strength. A restriction to this technique is that there are mRNAs that have no poly(A) tail. The yield of total RNA is approximately 1 mg of total RNA per mg of fresh cardiac tissue. It is less in elastic arteries that contain much more connective tissue and fewer cells.

Quantification of abundant mRNAs

The quantitation of mRNAs is based on the hybridization of a single mRNA species to a specific radioactive probe, and then the identification and quantification of the hybrid by electrophoresis followed by autoradiography. The most commonly used techniques to quantitate nucleic acids, including DNA and RNA, are called *Southern* and *Northern blot analysis*. Southern blot was historically the first technique and was developed by P. Southern to analyze DNA cut into fragments of manageable size. Northern was intended as a pun and now refers specifically to mRNA analysis. DNA fragments or mRNAs are fractionated by electrophoresis, transfered to a nitrocellulose or nylon membrane by capillarity and then exposed to a specific radioactive probe. The probe hybridizes to the homologous DNA fragment or mRNA; the unhybridized probe is then removed by washing with buffers of increasing stringencies; finally the radioactive hybrid is identified by autoradiography and quantified by scanning (Fig. 1. 13).

When the appropriate conditions of stringency are well determined, it is possible to apply total RNA directly onto a membrane without electrophoresis. This so-called slot or dot blot analysis is rapid and allows an absolute quantification of a given mRNA by depositing known amounts of sense RNA as a standard directly to the membrane [Mondry et al. 1995]. Results are usually expressed as a relative amount of a given mRNA to either the 18S fraction of ribosomal RNA that has been radioactively probed, or the total poly(A) containing sequences that represent the total mRNAs, or, like for PCR, another mRNA that is known to be unaffected by the experimental procedure.

To study shifts in isogene expression or to analyze the expression of isogenes or genes that belong to the same family, requires special care since these nucleotide sequences are highly homologous. When it is impossible to obtain a specific probe for each isoform, one needs to use other more specific techniques such as S1 nuclease, RNase protection assays (see below), or PCR.

Quantification of rare mRNAs.

Membrane proteins, receptors, regulatory peptides all belong to this group of mRNAs. Several methods can been used to study these mRNAs. The mRNA concentration can be increased, as previously explained. It is now preferable to utilize PCR or RNase protection.

S1 nuclease assay and the RNase protection assay consists of making a DNA-RNA hybrids for the first technique or an RNA-RNA hybrid for the RNase protection and to hydrolyze the single strands of DNA or RNA with S1 nuclease or RNases. One uses large quantities of total RNA (100 to 200 μg which represents 100 to 200 mg of myocardium, for example) in a dilute solution. The S1 nuclease or RNases will digest all mismatched hybrids, which have single-stranded regions. The probe used for S1 nuclease is a complementary cDNA probe, the same that used for a Northern blot. RNases protection utilises an antisense-RNA transcribed in the test-tube, as above. These techniques can be recommended for detection of isoforms, or homologous sequences, since both S1 nuclease and the RNases are extremely sensitive tools and will digest mismatched hybrids even if the single strand nonhybridized regions is one nucleotide length. One must be aware, however, that these two techniques are rather time consuming.

Working with DNA

Working with DNA is much easier since environmental DNases are less abundant and active than RNases.

cDNA amplification
This is certainly the first technique that should be learned by people who want to start molecular biology even at an embryonic level. The technique uses bacteria as a tool (Figure 1. 17). DNA amplification is an absolute must and is the technique required to make the probe of interest in a sufficient amount for making experiments on a large scale. It is so simple that any physiologist will learn it quickly.

The fragment of interest that has to be amplified is introduced into a plasmid and is called an *insert*. The plasmid into which an insert has been introduced is now called a *recombinant plasmid*. The plasmid is commercially available and is a piece of bacterial DNA that behaves like an independent minichromosome. It contains a gene conferring resistance to an antibiotic, such as amplicilline or tetracycline. The plasmid is introduced into permeabilized bacteria and replicates by itself and the gene conferring resistance to the antibiotic is transcribed and translated. Only the bacteria containing the recombinant plasmids are resistant to the antibiotic added to the medium and survive. They all contain the same recombinant plasmids. It is possible to multiply bacteria until we obtain enough material. Techniques to purify plasmids from bacterial DNA are easily available. They belong to the routine techniques that do not require specialists or well-trained microbiologists.

Making a DNA library .

This technique is more difficult (Figure 1. 18) and is to be handled by more experienced workers. A DNA library is so called because it produces different DNA fragments available and ready to be isolated. Figure 1. 17 shows how the DNA of interest is selected. Let us follow one of the numerous protocols available, that used by F. Soubrier [1988] to isolate the gene encoding the rat angiotensin I converting enzyme (ACE) which is a protease responsible for the making of angiotensin II, a major determinant of arterial pressure. They first partially sequenced the protein, and, by using the genetic code (Table 1. 2), they synthesized the corresponding oligonucleotides. A cDNA library was then constructed from mRNAs isolated from endothelium, which is the tissue that contains the converting enzyme. The oligonucleotides are so specific that they can only hybridize to the DNA fragments of the library that contain the corresponding gene products. It is then possible to isolate the spot that contains the hybrid, and then to reintroduce this spot into bacteria for amplification.

One of the techniques used to make the library is described in Figure 1. 18. The starting material is a mixture of cDNA fragments that is copied

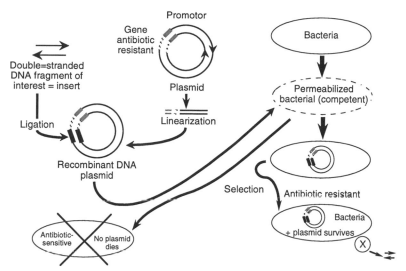

Fig. 1.17. Cloning and amplification [from Swynghedauw et al., 1993, with permission from Cardiovasc. Res. 27, 1566]

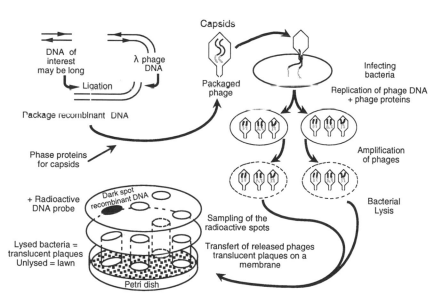

Fig. 1.18. DNA library using λ phage [from Swynghedauw et al., 1993, with permission from Cardiovasc. Res. 27, 1566]

from all the mRNAs present in the heart and that expresses, among other genes, the ACE. The ACE is a rather rare protein, and its mRNA is equally rare. In order to increase the chances to have a rat clone, the cDNA fragment is first introduced into bacteria by using phage transfection, which is more effective than plasmid transformation. The cDNA molecules are first ligated to a λ *phage DNA* to make a recombinant DNA. Then the recombinant DNA is packaged into *capsids* to give infectious phages. Capsids have the properties to attach to bacteria and to inject their DNA into the bugs, where it replicates and destroys the bacteria. The lysed bacteria release more phages, which infect more bacteria, and so on. On the Petri dish, lysed bacteria appear as translucent plaques and unlysed bacteria appears as a lawn. The released material is then transfered to a nitrocellulose membrane, and DNA is hybridized to the radioactive oligonucleotide probe. The radioactive spot is then aligned with the corresponding plaque still containing many phages, all with the same insert.

Another approach consists of making radioactive antibodies against the corresponding peptide. It is then necessary to use phages capable of inducing the expression of the DNA that was incorporated. The cDNAs are ligated after a promotor in the λ phage, and the transfected bacteria can express the recombinant proteins. The plaques can now be screened with an antibody against the peptide of interest. The unique recombinant phage from a single plaque is reintroduced into bacteria so that we can collect enough DNA to subclone the insert in plasmids. New phages have been developed that also infect bacteria, but it is possible to recover plasmids directly from the bacteria.

DNA sequencing

The chemical method of Maxam and Gilbert was the most popular for a rather long period of time. Nevertheless, DNA sequencing is now performed using automatic sequencers, there are now sequencers available in every center, and knowledge of the details of the technique is now unnecessary for cardiologists. Such a technique is incredibly rapid as compared to amino acid sequencing and allows the sequencing of most of the genes and consequently of the proteins during a short period of time. There are now enzymatic techniques of sequencing that allow serial analysis of sequences unlimited in length, like those provided by the SAGE (see below).

GENE TRANSFERS

Gene transfer is the possibility to incorporate new genetic material into a cell where it can be expressed either as extrachromosomal material or after being incorporated into chromosomal DNA. The process occurs naturally during a viral infection by a retrovirus: nevertheless, it is also possible to produce gene transfer experimentally by injecting genetic material into isolated cells or even into adult tissues. Transgenic technology is a third possibility and consists of transferring genes into gametes to produce strains expressing the new DNA sequences.

Gene transfer during viral infection

Virus are living elements without nuclei and nuclear membrane and whose genetic material consists of either RNA or DNA. Retroviruses are RNA viruses whose genetic material is incorporated into the host's genome during infection (Fig. 1. 19). The infection process is initiated by an interaction with the viral envelope proteins and receptor molecules located on the plasma membrane of the cell to be infected. This interaction is followed by the internalization and uncoating of the virus. Hence, the retrovirus cycle includes a step during which the RNA is retrotranscribed into a double-stranded DNA and is further included into the host genome using a second virally encoded integrase. The new integrated viral material is called a

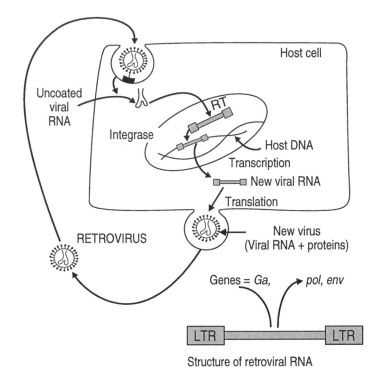

Fig. 1.19. The retrovirus cycle

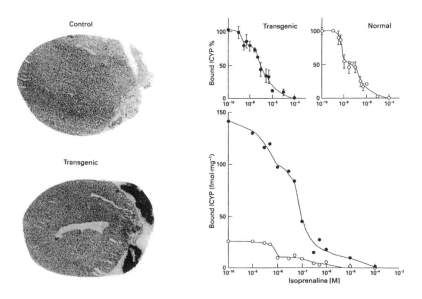

Fig. 1.20. Overexpression of human β1–AR in transgenic mice [from Bertin et al. 1993, with permission]

provirus and has the structure LTR-genes-LTR. The *long terminal repeats* (*LTR*) regions of the provirus regulate the expression of the viral gene and include *viral promoter,* e*nhancer* and *polyadenylation sequences.* LTR result from the duplication of terminal sequences during the retrotranscription. Genes, in the LTR-genes-LTR structure, include genes that allow complete replicaton of the virus and encode reverse transcriptase, integrase (*pol*), the viral core (*gag*), and the viral membrane (*env*) (names of the genes are usually printed in *italic*). Subsequently, the viral material is transcribed, and new virus particles are produced and exit the cell. The process does not harm the host cells.

During these steps, both the host's genome and the viral genome may acquire new DNA sequences, which, in a sense, perverts the transfected genome, which, in turn, can become transformant. Such a concept is one basis for the oncogenic theory of cancer. Retroviruses includes HIV, which is the virus responsible for AIDS. It is also very likely that the process of retrovirus infection may have played a role during evolution and that, for example, we acquired some viral sequences of interest by using this procedure (such as intronless genes encoding the adrenergic receptors).

Transgenic technology

Techniques

Transgenic animals are becoming a new tool accessible to physiologists and pharmacologists. There are now both a number of transgenic animals commercially available (as the transgenic strains of hypertensive rats) and several companies that generate transgenic strains to researchers. The most commonly used technique relies on direct injection of the DNA of interest into the male pronucleus of fertilized eggs from mice. The injected embryos are then reimplanted in a pseudopregnant foster mother and allowed to develop to term (Figure 1. 20). The resulting pups are screened to detect those animals that have incorporated the injected DNA in their genome. DNA is prepared from the tail or ear of the transgenic mice and analyzed by Southern blot. In experienced hands, the injected DNA is usually found in 25% of the pups. To be useful for physiological or pharmacological studies, the foreign gene must be expressed as an mRNA and a protein in the relevant organ. In terms of altered functional activity, the final yield may be extremely low and the financial cost very high.

The microinjected DNA can be an entire gene, including its own promotor, but usually it is a chimeric construct consisting of a tissue-specific promotor and the coding (or noncoding, if we want to specifically block - geneticists say to *knock out* - gene expression) part of a gene not usually controlled by the selected promotor. Three different aspects of transgenic technology have been applied to cardiovascular research [reviewed in Swynghedauw 1996].

(1) One of the goals is to target gene expression to a specific part of the cardiovascular system. By so doing, we want to overexpress or to suppress the expression of a gene, with the hope of altering the corresponding cardiac or vascular function and practicing what we may call *reverse physiology*. To attain such a goal, the choice of the promotor is of crucial importance, and it is now possible, for example, to target expression specifically to the myocardium as opposed to the coronary vessels. For example, the promotor controlling the transcription of the atrial natriuretic factor (ANF) gene is constitutively active only in the atrium (see Chapter 2) and can be used to target the expression of any coding sequence to this part of the heart (Field 1993, Bertin et al. 1993). The promotors of the ventricular myosin light chain 2 or α-myosin heavy chain are active only in the ventricles; that of vasopressin directs gene expression in the anterior pituitary and the pancreas while that of neurofilament F is specific for the pituitary. Hence any coding DNA controlled by these promotors will be transcribed only in the tissue in which the promotor is functional. It is also

possible to use nonspecific promotors, such as the metallothionein promotor and, by chance, get specific cardiac expression (Table 1. 3).

Table 1. 3. Cardiovascular specific promoters [references are in Swynghedauw 1996]

Tissue & Gene	Specificity	Activity
Atria		
Atrial natriuretic factor	+++	+
Ventricles + Atria		
α-myosin heavy chain	++	+++
Ventricles		
Myosin light chain 2_V	+++	++
Ventricles + Skeletal muscle		
β–Myosin heavy chain	++	+++
Creatine kinase	+	+
Myosin light chain 2_f	++	++
α–skeletal actin	++	+++
Myoglobin	++	++
Vessels		
α-1(I) collagen	±	++
α-smooth actin	++	++
Endothelin-1	+++	+

Our main point of interest here is the gene product itself. It could be the coding part of the selected gene controlled by its own promotor if the entire genomic sequence is injected. But then its expression will be regulated as is the endogenous gene, and there will be no advantage in using transgenic mice. Usually the goal is to take advantage of a tissue-specific promotor to overexpress or to inhibit the expression of a chosen protein. One good example is the pioneer work of L. Field [1993] who obtained an arrhythmogenic atrial tumor in transgenic mice by injecting a chimeric gene consisting of the ANF promotor and the coding region of an oncoprotein. In our laboratory, we have developed a new transgenic model of atrial β1-adrenoceptor overexpression [Bertin et al. 1993; Figure 1. 20]. In this model, the expression of the adrenergic receptors has been targeted to the atria by using the ANF promotor sequence, instead of the naturally occurring promotor of the receptor gene, and the purpose of the experiment was to modify the normal b1-adrenergic/muscarinic receptor ratio of atria, and more particularly of the cells of the sinus node, to modify the normal regulation of the heart rate and to change heart rate variability, a parameter of crucial importance for predicting sudden death in clinical cardiology. The result of this reverse physiology was a disappearance of heart rate variability in transgenic strains, which demonstrates that the atrial phenotype, in terms of autonomous system components, is as important as baroreflexs or central nervous system influences.

Another interesting approach consists of injecting an antisense mRNA to block the expression of the normally occurring mRNA. For example, Pepin et al. [1992] impaired the glucocorticoid feedback loop of ACTH synthesis and secretion by injecting into the fertilized egg a construct consisting of the neurofilament F promotor controlling the transcription of an RNA complementary to a portion of the 3' noncoding region of the rat glucocorticoid receptor cDNA.

This antisense RNA has minimal sequence homology with other members of the steroid hormone receptor gene superfamily, but it hybridizes specifically to the glucocorticoid receptor type mRNA and inhibits its expression. Consequently, the transgenic mice becomes obese and exhibits very high plasma levels of ACTH and corticosterone while the glucocorticoid maximal binding capacity of the pituitary was greatly diminished. Several other examples are given Tables 1. 4 and 1. 5.

(2) An entirely different strategy consists of analyzing the promotor. A construct is made with the promotor of interest linked to a *reporter*, which is a gene encoding an easily scorable protein to monitor the activity of the promotor. Most of the reporter genes code for enzymes not expressed in the tissue where the promotor is active, such as the bacterial enzyme chloramphenicol acetyltransferase, never present in mammalian organs, or β-galactosidase, normally present only in the gut. Even more elegant is the

Table 1. 4. Transgenic models of cardiac hypertrophy and failure [references are in Swynghedauw 1996]

Genetic construct (promoter) : *coding*	Resulting phenotype

Overexpression of transcription factors.

Protooncogenes

(RSV-LTR) : *c-myc*	Mild hyperplasia of cardiocytes
	Cardiac hypertrophy
	⇑ T3-induced myocyte growth
p21 c-ras	Hypertrophy + diastolic dysfunction
v-fps (tyrosine kinase)	Cardiac fibrosis + hypertrophy
IL-6+IL-6R	Cardiac hypertrophy
	+ impaired relaxation

Skeletal factors

(Moloney LTR) : *bmyf5*	Hypertrophy (4 chambers)
MyoD	Heart Failure + shortened lifespan
	Fibrosis, Skeletal proteins (patchy area)

Viral transcription factors

(Metallothionein 1) : *PVLT*	Cardiomyopathy + Enormous heart
(β-MHC) : *tsA58*	Cardiac & skeletal myopathy
(ANF) : *SV40 T antigen*	Atrial tumor, arrhythmias
(α-MHC) : *SV40 T antigen*	Hyperplastic atria & ventricles
	+ Ventricular arrhythmias
EBNA-LP	Dilated cardiomyopathy

Overexpression of adrenergic receptors.

(ANF) : *β1-AR*	No hypertrophy
(α-MHC) : *β2-AR*	No hypertrophy
(α-MHC) : *α1B-AR*	Hypertrophy + ⇑ ANF in ventricle

Others

(ANF) : *calmodulin*	Hyperplasia
MHC mutations	Cardiac hypertrophy
	+ Outflow tract gradient

---

use of a reporter gene coding for a secreted protein such as human growth hormone wthat can be directly measured in the blood of transgenic mice by radioimmunoassay.

This very common use of chimeric promotor-reporter gene constructs has been used to identify the DNA sequences that regulate the activity of a promotor after hormonal treatment, during differentiation or after mechanical stretch for example. It has also been used in cardiology to try to identify the regulatory regions sensitive to mechanical overload [Chien 1990].

(3) The mouse is the commonly utilized animal species for very practical reasons: it is inexpensive, it is very fertile, the gestation is short and it matures at an early age (3 weeks) so that one can obtain transgenic mice rapidly. ECG and hemodynamic studies are now possible in mice that beat at 500 bpm and have a predominant sympathetic tone [reviewed in

Swynghedauw 1996]. Transgenic models of hypertension have also been developed in rats that facilitates the measurement of blood pressure since the tail-cuff method has not been yet adapted to mice. Another approach is the use of transgenic pigs to make up xenografts (and also human blood) - that is to use animals organs that have been rendered tolerant to human immune system by transgenic technology for transplantations.

Gene transfer using transgenic technology is a random process, and there is evidence to suggest that the resulting phenotype may also depend on the location of the newly transfered constructs into the overall genome. Such an inconvenience could be overcome by the use of gene targeting in mouse embryonic stem cells. This is a new, time-consuming technique that provides the means to generate mice of any desired genotype [Capecchi 1989; Kurihara et al. 1994]. For the moment, transgenic technology is probably more useful as a tool for experimental research or pharmacology, mainly because it allows one to study the physiological properties of a species or organ in which known changes in genetic expression have been induced.

Table 1. 5. Exploring the myocardial function using transgenic technology [references are in Swynghedauw1996]

Myocardial dysfunction	Genetic construct (promoter) : *coding*
Electrical properties	
⇓ Heart Rate Variability + ⇑ contractility	(ANF) : *β1-AR*
+ no effect of iso + no arrhythmias	
⇑ AP duration + ⇑ diastolic $(Ca_{2+})_i$	*Cardiac overexpression of Na/Ca exchanger*
Lusitropism	

⇑ relaxation velocity + ⇑ contractility + no inotropic effect of iso + ⇑ Ca affinity of SR CaATPase	*Targeted disruption of phospholamban*
⇑ Time to half relaxation ⇓ Contractilité Diastolic dysfunction + ⇓ α-TM	(α-MHC) : *MLC2v* ⇑ *MLC2v in atria only* *Overexpression of β-TM*

Inotropism

⇓ contractility + ⇓ systolic Ca level + ⇓ decreased SR Ca transport	(αMHC) : *Phospholamban*
⇑ contractility + ⇑ heart rate + ⇑ basal Adenylate Cyclase + no effect of iso	α-MHC : β2-AR
⇓ iso-induced inotropism ⇑ ino and chronotropic effects of iso, fibrosis with aging	*β–AR kinase* $G_s\alpha$

Tolerance to ischemia

⇑ tolerance to zero-flow ischemia	(Cytomegavirus enhancer + β-actin promoter) : *HSP70*

Transgenic models of cardiac hypertrophy and failure

The most common cause of cardiac hypertrophy is mechanical overload, and several studies have suggested that the first biological events that link the overall activation of protein synthesis to mechanical stretch are an increased expression of several growth signals, including oncoproteins, growth factors, or nuclear transcription factors, or activation of several tranduction pathways, such as an enhanced production of IP3 or cAMP. Nevertheless, there also convincing evidences that mechanical overload is accompanied by an activation of autocrine systems as endothelin or angiotensin production [Yamazaki et al. 1996]. Transgenic technology was utilized to hierarchize these different levels of expression and succeeded in creating transgenic models of cardiac hypertrophy by using tumorigenic oncoproteins or nuclear transcription factors. Cardiac hypertrophy was also obtained using several transgenic manipulations that were not directly oriented to this purpose (Table 1. 4).

The pioneer work was that of L. Field, who succeeded in generating a transgenic mice model with atrial tumour and arrhythmias, this was obtained by targeted expression of a viral oncoprotein, the SV40 large T-antigen, and using the ANF promoter. Such an experiment has definitely ruled out the dogma that the cardiocytes are terminally withdrawn from the cell cycle. The approach was not *stricto sensu* related to cardiac hypertrophy; nevertheless, this work was at the origin of most of the transgenic study related to cardiac pathology. The disguised proliferative capacity of adult cardiocytes from murines has also been demonstrated by generating transgenic mice with different promoters. By 21 days of age many of these animals also exhibited gross cardiac pathology with a bilateral atrial hyperplasia, predominantly in the right atria, arrhythmias, and also a ventricular involvement with mitotic cardiomyocytes containing the T-antigen.

Cardiac hypertrophy has first been initiated by using several types of transcription factors, such as, for example, *c-myc,* a nuclear protooncogene that is activated during the early stage of mechanical overload [Bauters et al. 1988]. A 20-fold increase in *c-myc* expression was obtained by transgenic technology using an active, although nonspecific, promoter, and is accompanied by a doubling in the number of cardiocyte. Transgenic mice have a bigger heart (46%) and myocyte hyperplasia. It also enhances the growth response of the heart to isoproterenol and the thyroid hormone. A model of cardiac fibrosis has been proposed using *v-fps*, another oncogene. Ventricular hypertrophy was also associated with a ventricular overexpression of *p21 ras*, Interleukin-6, IL-6, and IL-6 receptor. Specific cardiac myogenic regulators are for the moment a rather controversial issue. Skeletal myogenic regulators, such as *bmyf5* and *MyoD*, were utilised and expressed into the heart by using strong nonspecific promoters. The cardiac expression of these regulators give rise to ectopic expression of the skeletal contractile proteins, cardiac hypertrophy, and evidence of congestive heart failure.

A model that associates both cardiac and skeletal myopathy, and as such resembles to some muscular dystrophies observed in human, was achieved in mice by targeting the simian virus tsA58 to the heart and skeletal muscles by using the promoter of the β-MHC. The same type of results was obtained using an early gene of polyomavirus, large T-antigen (PVLT), or the Epstein-Barr virus nuclear antigen-leader protein (EBNA-LP). Several genetic manipulations at this level have lethal consequences. The topic is of interest for the understanding of congenital cardiopathy. The *Sox* gene family plays an important role during embryogenesis. The targeted disruption of *Sox-4* generates homozygous embryos that succumb to cardiac failure at day 14 with an impaired development of the endocardial ridges into the semilunar valves and the septum resembling the common arterial trunk in clinic [references are in Swynghedauw 1996]. Transgenic expression of protooncogenes such as *c-myc*, *c-ras*, or *c-fps*, that are oncogenes activated by cardiac mechanical overload, usually induces a form of cardiac hypertrophy that is well-tolerated. In contrast, the cardiac expression of exogenous transcription factors, either of viral or skeletal origin, has pronounced deleterious effects.

Mechanical factors are undoubtedly at the origin of cardiac hypertrophy: nevertheless, it is also welldocumented that several hormones may also play a role, even in conditions as hypertensive cardiopathy. Converting enzyme inhibition prevents cardiac hypertrophy and myocardial fibrosis, and there is convincing evidences that such effects were related to both the reduction of the afterload and a specific trophic effect. Several hormonal or peptide stimuli are known to activate transcription and to stimulate myocardial growth both in an exocrine and in an autocrine fashion, including angiotensin II, endothelin I, and also β- and α1-adrenergic agonists. Nevertheless, *in vivo* experiments trying to evidence a trophic effect of these agents are confounded by concomitant peripheral effects on vasomotricity. Several types of approaches have been developed to study such a signalling pathways. In brief, the targeted overexpression of β1- or β2-AR unexpectedly did not induce cardiac hypertrophy. In contrast, the cardiac-specific overexpression of the α_{1B}-AR evidenced cardiac hypertrophy and activates the phospholipase C pathway.

Calmodulin is developmentally regulated, and calmodulin levels decline during the early postnatal stages in close association with the diminishing population of proliferative cardiocytes, suggesting that calmodulin may influence myocyte proliferation. A targeted model with a cardiac overexpression of calmodulin produced exaggerated cardiac growth response. Calmodulin is likely to play a critical role in initiating protein synthesis, as several classes of calmodulin antagonists reversibly blocked this process in Ehrlich ascites tumor cells. This article was the first to involve calmodulin into the cardiac growth process.

Familial hypertrophic cardiomyopathy (FHC) is an important clinical subject (see Chapter 4). FHC is linked to several mutations located into several contractile proteins. A transgenic strain with MHC mutations has recently arisen, evidencing cardiac hypertrophy with an outflow tract gradient. The mutant protein acts as a dominant negative and constitutes only 10% of the total myosin in the myocardium. In addition, while the trangene is expressed in the four chambers, only the left ventricle demonstrates enlargement, suggesting that hypertrophy needs to become a salient feature of hemodynamic factors.

Transgenic models of cardiac dysfunction

The targeted expression, or disruption, of genes that play a determinant role in myocardial functioning is a rather new challenge for cardiovascular physiologists (Table 1. 5). The first results of these genetic manipulations have generally confirmed what we already knew concerning several genes of crucial importance: phospholamban is indeed associated with relaxation and sensitive to isoproterenol, the β1-AR and β2-AR are determinants of the contractile state and heart rate and the heat shock proteins participate in the preconditioning. The second rather unexpected result was that mice survive after the disruption or overexpression of genes encoding proteins of crucial importance for the myocardial function, such as phospholamban, β-AR or Na/Ca exchanger, suggesting that the genetic transfer induces compensatory mechanisms. The combination of these two groups of results brings new informations about the real protein function *in situ* - that is not only on the direct effects of the protein, such as an effect on contractility of the adrenergic receptors, for example, but also on the indirect function of the same protein as a member of a transregulation system, at the level of the muscarinic system for example, which is usually unexplored.

A study from the group of Evangelia Kranias has investigated the effects of targeted disruption of the gene encoding phospholamban (PL) (see Chapter 2). It was not surprising to see that the disruption of the PL gene activates relaxation, increases the affinity for calcium of the Ca^{2+}ATPase, and suppress the effects of isoproterenol. Contraction was also activated, demonstrating that the two partners, contraction and relaxation, are linked together. In contrast, the targeted overexpression of PL gave rise to a phenotype that was roughly opposite and includes an unchanged heart size, a decrease in systolic calcium levels and shortening velocity, and a depressed basal systolic function. These differences were abolished on isoproterenol stimulation and due to an inhibition of the calcium transport function of the sarcoplasmic reticulum.

The physiologic function of myosin light chains (MLC) is still debatable. They certainly do not regulate the enzymatic activity of myosin and are likely to play a mechanical both at the level of the myosin hinge and actin binding site. The targeted overexpression of the MLC_{2v} results in overexpressing the transcript into ventricles and in expressing it into the atria, which do not normally contain this isoform. Using an isolated working heart preparation, the authors found that such a shift into atria severely affects contractile function and above all induces diastolic dysfunction with a slowed relaxation, suggesting that the atrial change has direct consequences on diastolic function or may reflect, as previously suggested, compensatory mechanisms that come into play in response to the transgenic modification. The same consequence on cardiac diastole was also obtained by overexpressing the β subunit of tropomyosin. The overexpression of one of the two subunits has also another consequence, which is a decrease in the cardiac content of the other isoform - namely the α-tropomyosin, which evidences, again and as above, a coordinate regulatory mechanism between the two tropomyosin isoform.

Gene transfer in autosomal cells

Pionner studies have been carried out by J.A. Wolff et al. [1990] on skeletal muscle and by E. Nabel [1989] on blood vessels. Transfer of a genetic construct was obtained by injecting pure RNA or DNA directly into the quadriceps muscles of mice. A significant protein expression of the reporter genes was then obtained *in situ* and maintained for at least 2 months [Wolff et al. 1990]. Porcine endothelial cells expressing recombinant b-galactosidase, a protein encoded by a reporter gene, from a retroviral vector, were introduced with a double balloon catheter into a denuded ilio-femoral artery, and 2 to 4 weeks later, it was shown that the β-galactosidase was reexpressed throughout the entire arterial endothelium, indicating that the DNA has been successfully transfected into the vessel wall (Nabel et al. 1989).

Striated muscles, such as myocardium, have a particular ability to efficiently express injected genetic constructs as compared to other tissues. Genetic constructs, including a reporter gene (such as CAT or luciferase) and a promotor, such as the Rous sarcoma virus promotor or the a-cardiac myosin heavy chain promotor, were directly injected into the myocardium after thoracotomy in dogs and in rats [von Harsdorf et al. 1993; Buttrick et al. 1992]. The activity of the reporter genes was detectable in a 1 to 2 mm area around the injection site and was still detectable in 30% of the animals one month after injection. The viral promotor was more active than the cardiac-specific sequences. This technique is useful for studying the regulation of expression of a promoter, but the geographic extension of the infection is rather limited. Nevertheless this approach has been proposed to treat skeletal muscle myopathies by multiple injections of a material containing the nondefective gene.

For the cardiovascular system, we need a more systemic technique, and it has been proposed to intravenously inject the DNA construct by utilizing a vector such as a adenovirus [Stratford-Perricaudet et al. 1992] or an expression plasmid: cationic liposomes [Zhu et al. 1993]. Dose-response curves were obtained with efficient transfection even 9 weeks after injection in all the endothelial cells of the cardiovascular system and extravascular parenchymal cells with no treatment-related toxicity. The adenoviral construct is probably more efficient than other vectors including retroviruses, and it has been demonstrated that the viral DNA remains extrachromosomal.

These approaches are obviously preliminary experiments that precede gene therapy, and, for the moment, their practical utility is mainly to permit study of the mechanisms of regulation of genetic expression *in vivo* in adults.

GENOME-BASED METHODS

The entire sequence of mammalian genomes and at least that of several bacteria are expected to be accomplished within a few years. An enormous number of sequenced genes are now available in a database and accessible through the Internet, which allows identification of the sequences of interest through alignments on known sequences (see Table 1. 6). Internet cloning

Table 1. 6. Good adresses for Internet cloning: database informations

---

DNA sequences (EMBL/Genbank)

http://www.embl-heidelberg.de

http://www.ebi.ac.uk/ebi-home.html

There are also Sequence analysis and alignments; Cell and Molecular Biology Online....

Human Genome DataBase (GDB)

http://www.hgmp.mrc.ac.uk/

Molecular Biology Jump Station

http://www.horizonpress.com/gateway/molbiol.html

There are also PCR Jump Station, Genetics Jump Station.

Literature

Of course Medline: http/www.nlm.nih.gov

There is also The Internet Directory of BioTechnology Resources.

---

and bioinformatics are now full disciplines that have generated not only a new methodology but also a new form of biology, called *functional genomics*, as opposed to *structural genomics* [Hieter and Boguski 1997]. Functional genomics refers to experimental approaches that assess gene functions by using the informations provided by structural genomics. The fundamental new point is that functional genomics aims to study the entire function of a cell by analyzing the overall genetic expression of a given cell or organism. Most of these techniques are based on several assumptions that are detailed below. The most important of them is the fact that a short nucleotide sequence tag (9 to 10 bp) contains sufficient information to uniquely identify a mRNA n a large database.

Expressed sequence tags

Large-scale partial sequencing of cDNA libraries is now possible to use to discover novel genes and characterize transcriptional patterns in different tissues. The technique consists in using cDNA λ phage libraries and plating phage plaques (see Figure 1. 18) as a direct source of cDNA clones. Phage eluates were then used for PCR reaction using two standard primers. After amplification, PCR products were directly used as a template for fluorescent automated DNA sequencing. Partial cDNA sequences, also called *expressed sequence tags* (*EST*), are then used to retrieve entire sequences by various strategies from databases [Adams et al. 1991]. Mapping of EST to chromosomes is now rather a routine technique. The technique consists in screening series of somatic cell lines that contain defined sets of chromosomes for the presence of EST and then analyzing the segregation pattern of PCR products from hybrid DNA templates [Adams et al. 1991, Hwang et al. 1997]. Using such a strategy CC Liew's group in Toronto has published the first publicly available database of human cardiovascular containing 43,285 ESTs, of these 55% matched to known genes, 33% matched only to other ESTs, and 12% represented entirely novel and unknown transcripts [Hwang et al. 1997]. In addition, cardiovascular gene chromosome transcripts maps were generated by using a specific database and a sequence clustering algorithm. With such a protocol, 1,048 ESTs were localized to chromosomes. Comparisons between different fetal heart and adult heart libraries exhibited, for example, as expected, higher expression of genes involved in RNA and protein expression and lower expression of cell structure/motility in the fetus (22 to 33% and 14 to 18%) than in adult (12 to 17 and 22 to 25%). 34 genes were potentially overexpressed in a cardiac hypertrophy library, including mitochondrial genome transcripts, myosin light chain-2, brain natriuretic peptide, desmin, HSP70, superoxide dismutase, ANF, α-tropomyosin, and α-actin. Several unexpected genes were found to be also overexpressed in this condition, including ribosomal proteins, tissue inhibitors of metalloproteinase-4 and prostaglandin D synthases, strongly suggesting that the methodology holds tremendous potential for genome-wide research for novel genes involved in cardiac remodelling.

Differential gene expression

Differential gene expression is obviously essential for every pathological process including cardiac hypertrophy, inherited diseases, coronary restenosis and vascular remodelling. Ancient techniques, now abandoned, attempted to detect heterogeinity between various populations of mRNAs isolated, for example, from a normal and a hypertrophied heart by computer analysis of hybridization curves [de la Bastie et al. 1987], or by substractive library screening and differential hybridization using various pools of RNA or cDNA [Sambrook et al. 1989]. Similar techniques using PCR have recently been developed and termed *RNA display* [Liang and Pardee 1992]. They are presently extensively used to understand the molecular mechanisms involved in various cardiovascular diseases and to discover novel targets for pharmacological research or gene therapy [Wang and Feuerstein 1997] (Table 1. 7). These techniques have to be known even by the nonspecialist because they currently represent an essential tool for future research.

68

Table 1. 7. Distribution of genes in the human cardiovascular system [rearranged from Hwang et al. 1997].

Functional category	Number of known genes (and percentage)
Cell division (including apoptosis)	260 (5.68)
Cell signaling (including ion channels, receptors)	836 (18.27)
Cell structure and motility (including vesicular transport and contractile protein)	443 (9.68)
Cell defense (including immune system)	307 (6.71)
Gene expression (including RNA and protein expression)	1,097 (23,97)
Metabolism	717 (15.67)
Unclassified	915 (20.00)

mRNA differential display [Wang and Feuerstein 1997, Liang and Pardee 1992] is basically a three-steps procedure. Step one is a reverse transcription (RT) made on a large pool of DNA-free mRNAs extracted from the two tissues of interest (lets say a normal and a hypertrophied rat heart) and uses a set of 3' (or downstream)-anchored primers, so-called because they are made with a long T repeat (for example, 12 T - T_{12} -) which is complementary to the 3'-polyadenylated tail of mRNAs + two bases (Figure 1. 21).

The result of such a RT is already a first selection of mRNAs since the pool is made only with polyT-containing cDNAs, which represents most, but not all, of the eucaryotic mRNAs. Another selection comes from the fact that primers were made with four different bases at the last base of the 3'-end; such subgroups allows a portion of the RNA to be already

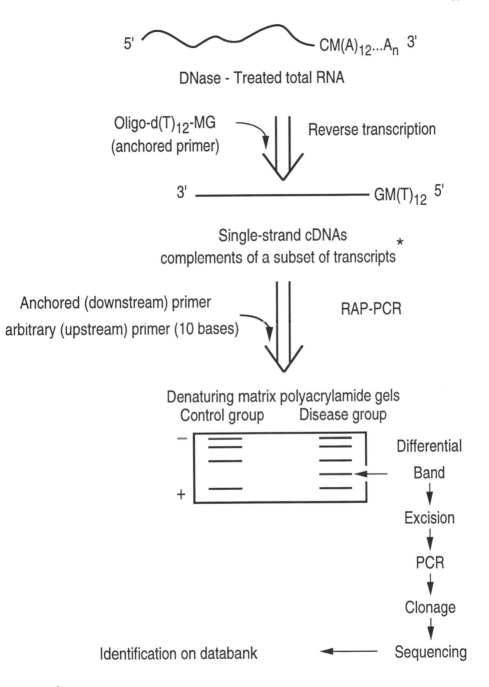

*4 Subgroups G, A, C, or T. Subgroup G is only figured.

Fig. 1.21.   RNA display

70

displayed. Step two is a RNA Arbitrary Primed PCR (RAP-PCR) amplification. The primers are the downstream anchored primers identical to that used for RT and arbitrary upstream primers which are usually 10 bases in length and composed of approximately 50% G+C and 50% T+A. It has been shown that at least 30 to 50 upstream primers will be necessary to amplify every mRNA species in a given tissue. Step three consists in resolving the amplified cDNA fragments by electrophoresis followed by

Table 1. 8. Examples of applications of mRNA differential displays to cardiovascular research (rearranged from Wang and Feuerstein 1997].

Source and function	Novel gene discovered
Heart	
Left ventricular overload	Several cytoskeletal proteins
Cardiac transplantation	Cell-surface receptors
	Allograft inflammatory factor-1
Carnitine-deficient heart	Carnitine Transferase
Vessels	
Oxidative stress response	Aldo reductase
Shear stress response	Cyclooxygenase, SO dismutase, NO synthase
IP-10	Endotoxin shock
Angioplasty	BART-1

autoradiographic detection. Up- or down-regulated gene (or more frequently gene fragments) can then be detected, recovered, subcloned (that is purified), sequenced, and, based on the sequence information, identified by using a computer database (Internet cloning). The fulllength cDNA clone can then be isolated by screening a cDNA library, and the protein can be deduced from the DNA sequence. The technique has already allowed the discovery of several genes whose expression is related to the process of atherogenesis, diabetes, cardiac overload (Table 1. 8).

The serial analysis of gene expression (SAGE)

SAGE does not belong *per se* to differential analysis techniques. SAGE allows the detailed analysis of thousands of transcripts (and then, if requested, the comparison between two different tissues, which is a differential analysis) after reverse transcription and is based on two principles [Velculescu and Zhang 1995] (Figure 1. 22). (1) A short nucleotide sequence tag (9 to 10 bp) contains sufficient information to uniquely identify a mRNA, provided it is isolated from a define position within the transcript. (2) Concatenation of short nucleotide sequences tag can be created by ligation and allows the efficient analysis of mRNAs in a serial manner by the sequencing of multiple tags within a clone. The sequencing of these multitags is now easy using enzymatic sequencing.

Cliveage of cDNA into smaller fragments is obtained in two steps by restriction endonucleases. These fragments are then oriented in a defined position by binding their 3' portion to streptavidin beds, divided in half, and ligated to one of two different linkers using a combination of anchoring and tagging enzymes to yield short sequence tags. Ditags are then formed by ligation and serve as templates for PCR amplification using two different primers specific for each of the two linkers. Cleavage of the PCR products with anchoring enzymes allowed isolation of ditags that are ready for concatenation.

The SAGE allowed, for example, comparisons between normal pancreas and colon and colon and pancreas tumors and provided the identification of 49,000 different genes. 54% of the tags matched Genbank

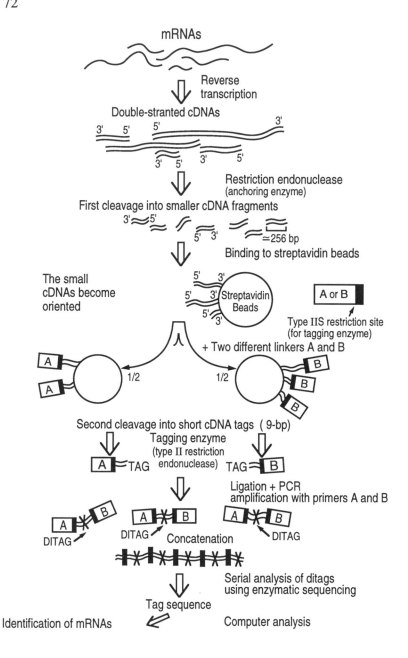

Fig. 1.22. Serial analysis of gene expression (SAGE)
[from Velculescu and Zhang 1995]

entries, the others were unidentified genes. Identified genes were mostly expressed at a rather high degree of abundancy (>500 copies per cell). When normal and cancer tissues were compared, 289 transcripts were expressed at different levels [Zhang et al. 1997].

DNA microarrays

DNA microarrays consisting of individual gene sequences printed in a high-density array on a glass microscope slide are now available in microbiology, for bacteria whose entire genome is already known [DeRisi et al. 1997]. Microarrays, containing approximately 6,400 distinct DNA sequences, were used to characterize the changes in genetic expression that take place for nearly the entire genome of yeast during the shift from anaerobic to aerobic metabolism. Glucose-depleted medium induced the expression of more than 700 genes by a factor of 2 and allowed the reconstruction of the cassical biochemical scheme for glucose induction in a complete different way, in addition, a large group of the genes are unknown. And this is just one example!

The technique has already been applied to humans, although we know only a limited amount of expressed genes [Schena et al. 1996]. Microarrays containing 1,046 human cDNAs were used to examine the heat-shock response (a topic of growing interest in molecular cardiology) in cultures human T cells. Comparative expression analysis of heat-shocked versus control cells revealed 17 diffrentially expressed genes, and sequence analysis had confirmed the validity of the technique by evidencing an enhanced expression of HSP-90. It also allowed the discovery of three new transcripts that did not match any entry in the public database. When the entire human genomic structure is known and such a technical approach is available for experimental medicine, the technological approach should even become much more rapid and paradoxically more simple.

THE NORMAL HEART AND VESSELS
MOLECULAR STRUCTURE IN RELATION TO PHYSIOLOGY

Our current understanding of the molecular structure of the heart and the vessels has considerably increased over the last several years. Nearly all of the genes coding for known cardiovascular proteins have been cloned and sequenced, and a considerable amount of orphan genes have been detected by using genome-based techniques (12% in [Hwang et al. 1997]). Information also has been obtained from genomic sequences that concern the regulatory parts of the genes and subsequently their potential physiological regulation. Obviously, such a topic may constitute an entire book. A selection has therefore been made among an enormous mass of information in order to retain the data that have potential interest in terms of physiological and pharmacological properties.

MEMBRANE PROTEINS AND ELECTRICAL ACTIVITY

Inter and intracellular cross-talk

Every cell possess external membranes, endoplasmic (sarcoplasmic in muscle) reticulum membranes, and nuclear membranes. The last two are internal membranes and, in part, responsible for intracellular compartimentation.

Table 2. 1. Main families or superfamilies of membrane proteins. The thyroid and steroid nuclear receptor superfamily are intranuclear transcription factors and, stricto sensu do not belong to membrane proteins. They have in common a ligand and a DNA binding domain with Zn finger dependent structure.

---

1. The R7G receptor family

7 transmembrane domains + G protein binding site

Adrenergic, muscarinic, dopaminergic, angiotensin II, bradykinin, endothelin receptors

2. The voltage-gated plasma membrane ionic channels

Several transmembrane domains containing 6 transmembrane helices, one helix (S4) is a voltage sensor, inactivation is controlled by a lid

Na^+ and Ca^{2+} channels

3. The P-type class of ATPases

Catalytic cycle that involves a phosphorylated protein intermediate, 10 transmembrane domains (still controversial)

Na^+, K^+ ATPase, plasma membrane calcium ATPase, calcium ATPase of the sarcoplasmic reticulum

4. Receptors with tyrosine kinase activity

Extracellular ligand binding domain, cytosolic tyrosine kinase activity, dimers or monomers active after dimerisation

PDGF, EGF, FGF, insulin receptors

5. Exchangers

12 transmembrane domains, use energy indirectly through the sodium gradient

Na^+/H^+ and Na^+/Ca^{2+} exchangers

The role of the external membrane is to maintain the polarity of the cell and transmit information coming from the environment. The transmission procedure is called *transduction*. The endoplasmic reticulum has to store rapidly available calcium within the cell. The role of the nuclear membrane is to isolate the genetic information from the cytoplasm, but there are numerous types of cells that do not have a nuclear membrane, and even in the heart the nuclear membrane is porous. Progress in genetic taxonomy (see Chapter 1. Gene and the genetic code. *Gene classification*) has simplified our current understanding of membrane proteins and allows a classification of membrane proteins that is based on structural and functional relationships (Table 2. 1).

The external membrane, or sarcolemma in the myocardium, is a phospholipid hydrophobic bilayer covered by glycoproteins (or glycocalyx) in which three groups of proteins are inserted - ion channels, receptors, and enzymes. Such a bilayer electrically isolates the cell from the extracellular space. This is the place where the cell receives external signals from other cells (Figure 2. 1). These signals are numerous and include hormones, ions, electrical currents, stretch, shear stress and growth factors. In addition, each signal acts through different targets - for example, norepinephrine binds to four different receptors. The multiplicity of intercellular signals is in contrast with the paucity of intracellular messengers that do not include more than 3 to 4 components including calcium (the most important messenger in muscles), cAMP, IP3, and diacylglycerol. Membrane proteins not only transduce the external signals into intracellular messenger but also sequentially amplify this information. In addition, intracellular messengers have diverse functions. For example, calcium not only couples mechanical contraction to excitation, but it also simultaneously activates calmodulin, and in turn at least 20 different enzymes.

78

A. Intercellular cross-talk

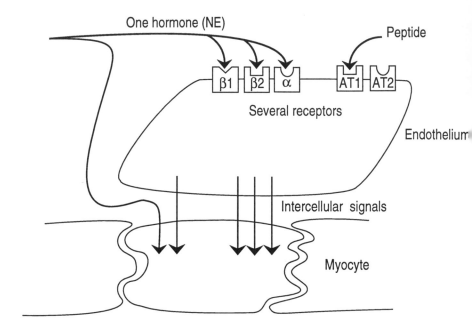

B. Intracellular messengers

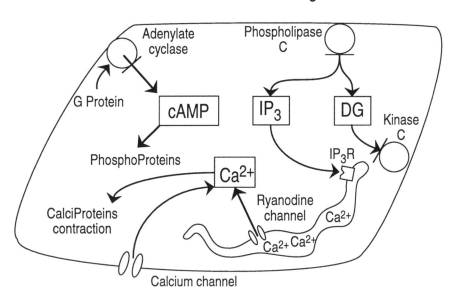

Fig. 2.1 Inter- and intracellular cross-talk

Receptors and receptology

Receptology is the most prominent branch of cardiovascular biology and pharmacology and thanks to bioinformatic, receptology, is now one of the main source of protein discovery. Studies on receptors now include not only the classical ligand binding but also a considerable amount of different techniques, including molecular biology, transgenic technology, and transfections.

Plasma membrane receptors and transduction systems

Stricto sensu, receptors are proteins that receive and transduce information, angiotensin II receptor subtype1 (AT1) binds angiotensin II (angio II) and by so doing knows that the vasculature needs to be vasoconstricted. Then, it activates the PI cycle and produces intracellular messenger such as IP3 that, in turn, may bind an IP3 receptor located on the endoplasmic reticulum inside the cell, which, in turn, will release calcium from the internal stores. Therefore, the role of AT1 is to transform a signal that is carried by a peptide, angio II, into another signal, chemically different and that has a broader and less specific field of activity.

Receptors not only transduce signals, but they also amplify the information. The β1-adrenergic receptor, β1-AR, binds epinephrine and by so doing knows that contractility has to be activated by exercising. Then the receptor binds and dissociates several G protein complexes that, in turn, liberate the $G_{\alpha s}$ subunits which in turn activate several molecules of adenylate cyclase, which produces several molecules of cAMP.

Classification of receptor families is actually based on structure and function relationships. Not all families play a significant role in the cardiovascular system, and this chapter deals only with those that really have a physiological effect in either myocardial or vascular physiology (Table 2. 1).

The R7 G family includes receptors that bind G proteins and possess seven hydrophobic spanning regions in their molecular structure [Strosberg 1987]. In addition, most are encoded by intronless genes. Most of the plasma membrane receptors of the cardiovascular system that have important physiological roles belong to this family. The agonists are compounds that are not soluble into the lipidic plamsa membrane bilayer, as opposed to ligand of nuclear receptors.

The β-adrenergic system consists of three elements, including a receptor, a coupling protein binding guanine nucleotides (G protein), and the adenylate cyclase. The phosphodiesterases that catalyze the hydrolysis of cAMP are not in a strict sense a part of the system but play a major role in the regulation of the physiological effects. The β-ARs (β2-AR is a glycoprotein, 64 kD) are wellcharacterized. Of importance for the physiologist is the presence of several consensus DNA sequences that play a regulatory role. These sequences include glucocorticoid, cAMP, and thyroxine responsive elements (GRE, CRE and TRE) all of which suggest hormonal control in the expression of the gene (Figure 2. 2). Every endocrinologist is indeed aware of the fact that, for example, thyrotoxicosis is accompanied by an increased sensitivity to catecholamines, which results from an overexpression of β-AR genes. The protein structure includes an extracellular N-terminal tail that binds glycoproteins, seven membrane-spanning regions that are arranged as a tunnel in which the agonist (or the β-agonist) binds, and a phosphorylatable C-terminal end that binds G protein.

The β2-AR receptor, as every receptor of the R7G family, is fully activated when it binds the corresponding hormone (although such a concept has been reconsidered based on transgenic data [Bond et al. 1995], see further) and then becomes able to interact with the heterotrimeric G protein

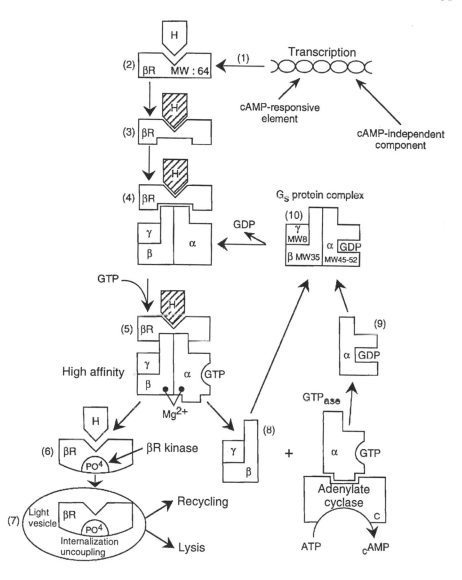

Fig. 2.2 The transduction system of the β-adrenergic receptors, β-R. Left: from β-R gene (1) to the internalized vesicles. Right: process of activation of the adenylate cyclase. H: hormone. α, β, γ: G protein subunits [from Swynghedauw 1990 with permission].

complex, leading to an exchange of the GDP previously bound to the G_{α}-subunit with GTP (Fig. 2. 2). The binding of GTP decreases the affinity of the receptor for the G protein and dissociates the G protein complex into α and $\beta-\gamma$ subunits. The α-GTP subunit then has the capacity to activate Adenylate Cyclase, or other effectors such as ionic channels. The α-subunit is also a GTPase, and the G protein complex needs to be reconstituted by GTP hydrolysis.

The cAMP concentration also depend on a membrane polymorphic enzyme, phosphodiesterase, which transforms the active nucleotide into AMP. The enzyme exists as several isoforms whose repartition varies in the heart and vessels and is inhibited by several compounds.

External receptors that belongs to this family can be internalized (Figure 2. 2) and inactivated, as a protection when the plasma concentration of the corresponding agonist is increased. This so-called homologous down-regulation is an extremely complex phenomena that may involve either a simple internalization of the receptor, which then becomes uncoupled from the transduction system, or an internalization followed by phosphorylation (by a specific β-adrenergic receptor kinase, Fig. 2. 2) and destruction, or even inhibition of transcription by a negative feed-back that utilizes the cAMP responsive element located on the gene. Conversely, prolonged treatment with a β-blocker upregulates the receptor and usually results in an increased receptor density.

Two transgenic models with a targeted overexpression of these two subtypes of AR have been reported. In the first model, a rather modest overexpression of the $\beta1$-AR overexpression has been induced into atria by using the promoter of ANF [Bertin et al. 1993, Mansier et al. 1996]. The heart rate was then monitored using telemetry and the signal was analyzed using a quantitative time-frequency domain analysis (the Wigner-Ville method). In the transgenic strain, heart rate was unchanged: nevertheless, the heart rate variability was hampered and the heart rate became insensitive to propranolol (Figure 1. 20). In addition, the basal level of atrial contractility was enhanced, and contractility was also insensitive to isoproterenol. In the second model [Milano 1994], a pronounced overexpression of the β2-AR was generated in the ventricles. These animals have a three times enhancement of the basal contractility which was equally unsensitive to isoproterenol. Therefore, whatever the degree of overexpression of β-ARs (8-fold in our study, 195-fold in the other), and whatever the β-AR subtype, the basal contractility is maximumly enhanced to an apparent saturation level.

New concepts concerning the receptors mechanism of action suggest that even in the absence of any agonist; a small fraction of the receptor pool is in an activated conformation [Bond et al. 1995]. Consequently any increase in the β-AR density will increase the absolute number of β-AR in active form. The number of activated receptors is then enhanced in the two transgenic mice strains (the β-ARs of these animals have indeed a very high affinity for the agonist [10^{-10} M] [Mansier et al. 1996]). Therefore, it is conceivable that the increase in β-AR density will maximally stimulate both the sinus node cells and cardiac myocytes. At the level of the sinus node, the heart rate cannot become faster because mice have a sympathetic tone, nevertheless it has lost the capacity to vary with normal physiological stimuli. At the level of the cardiocytes, basal atrial contractility is enhanced to a level that renders ineffective any addition of isoproterenol. The same rational is true for the β1- and β2-AR.

Transgenic manipulations were also made on regulatory elements of the adrenergic system. The β-AR kinase1 (β-ARK1) is a kinase that phosphorylates specifically the AR and by so doing participates in the processes of internalization of these receptors. Both the mRNA levels and the phosphorylation activity of the β-ARK1 are elevated in the human failing ventricles and participate in the down-regulation of the β-adrenergic receptors. A 3 to 5 fold increased expression of β-ARK1 has recently been obtained in mouse and has resulted, as expected, in a significant diminution of the isoproterenol-induced inotropic response [Koch et al. 1995], which was attributed to an increase rate of internalisation of the β-AR. A 3-fold overexpression of the transduction protein, $G_{s\alpha}$, was targeted to the heart [Iwase et al. 1996] with no changes in the adenylate cyclase activity or in the basal contractility of the heart. Nevertheless, the authors observed a phenotypic effect with an enhanced inotropic and chronotropic effect of isoproterenol as compared to controls. In addition, they also showed a toxic effect, analogous to the effect of chronic administration of catecholamines - namely, fibrosis [Iwase et al. 1996].

The adrenergic system comprises several receptors including β1 and 2, α1 and 2 and their subtypes. Recently a β3-subtype primarily expressed in the adipose tissue has been discovered, and a functional β3-AR coupled to Gi has been characterized in human heart and may modulate negative inotropic activity [Gauthier et al. 1996]. The system is a component of the autonomous nervous system (ANS) and, as such, is coupled with the muscarinic receptors. For the physiologist, the pathologist and the pharmacologist it is important to note that nearly every component of this system is polymorphic, inluding the receptors, α-subunits of the G proteins, adenylate cyclase (there are 7 isoforms of the cyclase and at least two are present in the heart), and phosphodiesterases (3 to 4 isoforms in the cardiovascular apparatus), resulting in infinite possibilities of regulation.

Figure 2. 3. is an attempt to reintegrate what is known about the ANS, from classical physiology and what we have recently learned from molecular biology. Both the sympathetic and the parasympathetic systems have a preganglionic step, a postganglionic step, a peripheral control, and finally physiological effects.

(1) In both cases acetylcholine and the corresponding acetylcholine nicotinic receptor mediates the transduction at the ganglionic level.

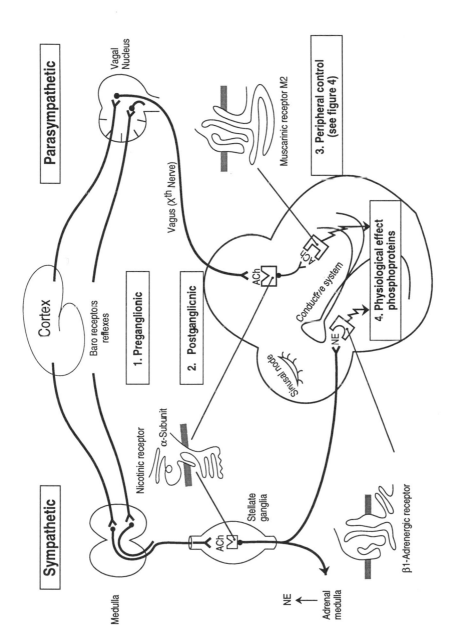

Fig. 2.3 Receptors of the cardiovascular autonomous nervous system

Nevertheless, this level is located in the stellate ganglions in the sympathetic cascade. By contrast, the ganglionic level of the parasympathetic system is located in the organ itself - that is around the sinus node and the auriculo-ventricular node. The nicotinic receptor has a 5-subunit stoichiometry and acts as an ionic channel (see below Ion channels and electrical activity).

(2)- The postganglionic neurones do not contain myeline, and release from their terminal varicosities either norepinephrine (NE) for the sympathetic system or acetylcholine for the parasympathetic system. These two neurotransmitters in turn act on specific receptors that are in the myocardium itself and belong to the R7G family - respectively, the β1-adrenergic receptor and the muscarinic receptor subtype M2.

(3) The receptors themselves are connected to a transduction system that includes the G proteins (Gs for the sympathetic and Gi for the parasympathetic systems), which are membrane proteins, the adenylate cyclases isoforms (V and VI are predominant in the heart, which also contains minor amounts of isoforms IV and VII), and the synthesis of cAMP. cAMP, in turn, binds cooperatively to two sites on the regulatory subunit of protein kinase A, releasing the active catalytic subunit (Figure 2. 2).

(4) Finally, the catalytic subunit of protein kinase A is translocated from its cytoplasmic and Golgi complex anchoring sites and triggers physiological activity by phosphorylating various phosphoproteins (on a serine in the context X-Arg-Arg-X-Ser-X), including troponin I, phospholamban and several ion channels but also transcriptional factors (see below in this chapter, Cardiac and vascular growth). Other receptors of the R7G family include dopaminergic receptors, angiotensin II, bradykinin, endothelin receptors.

G proteins

The G proteins are polymorphic membrane proteins that play a major role in controlling signal transduction. G proteins were discovered by the last two winners of the Nobel prize, Rodbell and Gilman [Gilman 1987] and are composed of three different polymorphic subunits, α, β, g, (MWs 45-52, 35 and 8 kd).

Molecular cloning has identified at least 20 different α-subunits. The αs-subunit isoforms are sensitive to cholera toxin and are encoded from splicing products of a single gene. They mediate the activation of adenylate cyclase and L-type calcium channels through the activation of β1-adrenergic, histamine, prostaglandin E2 and 5-HydroxyTyramine receptors. The αi-subunits 1, 2 and 3, but only αi2 and 3 are expressed in the heart, are sensitive to pertussis toxin and mediate adenylate cyclase inhibition and, in the sinus node, activation of the potassium channels. G proteins also mediate the regulation of the phosphoinositol pathway and the activation of phospholipase A2 through the activation of the other adrenergic receptors and also the angio II receptors.

Ion channels and electrical activity

Biological determinants of the action potential
Cells are polarized and the intracellular space, as compared to neutral, has a potential of -80 mV. Polarization is maintained by this ionic gradient. The intracellular K^+ concentration is higher (155 vs. 4 mM), and the Na^+ (12 vs. 145 mM), Cl^- (20 vs 123 mM) or Ca^{2+} (0.1 vs 1,500 microM) lower than in the extracellular space, conversely energy production (directly or indirectly) is required to release Na^+ or Ca^{2+} out of the cell or to allow K^+ to penetrate into the intracellular space.

These ionic movements create electrical currents whose intensity can be predicted from the ionic gradient according to Nernst's equation [Coraboeuf 1978]:

$$E_{ion} = (-62 \text{ mV}/z) \log([ion]_{in}/[ion]_{out}$$

z = ion valence and [ion] = ion concentration.

Current, I, can be directly measured using the patch-clamp technique. In this technique, a solution-filled micropipet connected to an amplifier is sealed onto the cell membrane. If an ion channel opens under the pipet, the current flowing across a single channel can be measured. Currents are expressed in amperes and are often described by Ohm's law:

$$I = V/R$$

V is voltage or driving force - that is the difference between the Nernst potential E_{ion} and membrane resting potential E_m. For example, the resting potential, - 80 mV, is close to E_K (- 90 mV) but not identical because there is still a certain degree of permeability for the Na^+ and Ca^{2+} ions at rest. Outward rectifying channels are channels that pass current more easily in the outward direction than another. Resistances are the transmembrane channels, which are holes in the membrane whose gating is commanded by voltage or hormones where R is the resistance of the channel to ion flow, $1/R$ is conductance (or permeability). The structure of these ionic channels is now known and structural/function relationships are rather wellestablished.

Action potential (AP (Figure 2. 4) is a passive event. It depends on an inward current due to the gating of a sodium channel and the passive influx of sodium. The opening of the channel itself is voltage-dependent and is triggered by a wave of depolarization that originates from the sinus node (conduction). The sodium current will in turn trigger the subsequent gating of a calcium current, which is also a passive event. The calcium channel is also a voltage-dependent ion channel. The cell is now fully polarized and even slightly hyperpolarized and needs to lose positive charges in order to recover its normal negative resting potential. These are again passive events due to the gating of a rather complex group of channels, potassium channels. The cell will then lose as many positive charges as were

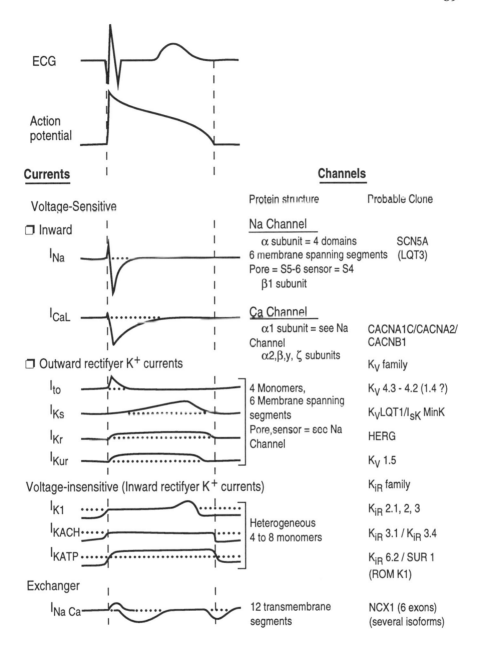

Fig. 2.4 The molecular basis of ECG

introduced by the sodium current, and at the end of the AP the cell will have recovered a potential of -80 mV. Nevertheless, it contains too much Na^+ and not enough K^+. The Na^+, K^+-ATPase, the so-called sodium pump, provides energy to reestablish the normal gradients and release sodium in exchange for potassium, and ATP consumption. Calcium has also to be released: this is the task of the Ca^{2+} ATPase of the sarcoplasmic reticulum and Na^+/Ca^{2+} exchange and Ca^{2+}ATPase of the external membrane.

ECG monitors the first derivative of the sum of all the AP of either the ventricles or the atria nevertheless, the shape of the ECG does also depend on various gradients across the myocardial wall (Figure 2. 4). In addition to the well-known modifications due to hypertrophy, ECG allows the measurement of the QT interval, which is of major prognostic value and represents the duration of the AP. Ischemia-induced elevation of the ST segment, for example, results from both a shortening of the AP and depolarization due to the loss of ATP when ischemia opens the ATP-dependent potassium channel. Depolarization is a consequence of both the intracellular loss of potassium and the accumulation of potassium in the extracellular space.

Figure 2. 4. tries to establish a bridge between what is currently known in clinical practice and both cellular physiology and molecular biology. The ECG corresponds to AP, and T wave indicates the repolarization process. On this figure, below AP, were schematically indicated currents, I, as obtained by potential steps triggering currents during voltage-clamp experiments. The currents are in amperes and on the drawing, inward currents are downward and outward currents upward. The addition of these currents gives rise to the AP. The right side of the figure shows the corresponding ion channels and some features concerning their protein and gene structure. The sodium current is due to the gating of the principal subunit of the sodium channel: the same is true for the calcium channels L (the most important) and T (which is specific for the conduction system).

91

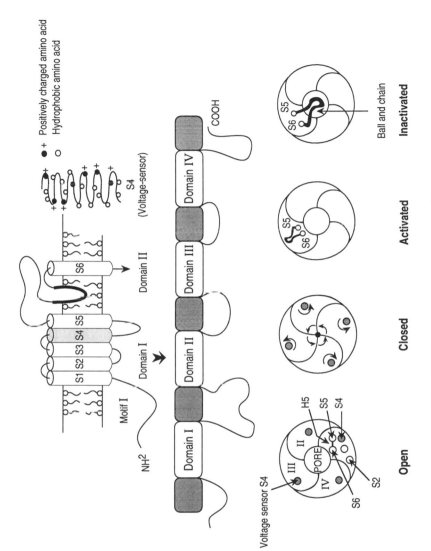

Fig. 2.5. The molecular structure of ion channels

Potassium channels are different since most of the potassium channels principal subunits all contribute to the formation of the pore as explained below.

Table 2. 2. Main ion channels of the cardiovascular system

---

1. Voltage-gated cation channels (except for conductive system): L-type Ca^{2+} channel, Na^+ channel, voltage-sensitive (outward rectifyer) K^+ channels (Kv)

2. Voltage-insensitive K^+ channels (inward rectifier, Kir): simple inward (background) rectifier K^+ channel, G-protein coupled muscarinic K^+ channel, ATP-sensitive K^+ channel

3. Anion channels: cystic fibrosis transmembrane conductance Regulator (CFTR) Cl^- channel, cAMP-activated Cl^- channel

4. Gap junctions: connexins (Cx 43) and connexons

5. Sinus node channels: T (predominant and specific of the sinus-node) and L-type Ca^{2+} channels, I_f (Na^+/K^+-dependent inward slowlydeveloping hyperpolarization-activated diastolic current), no Na^+ channel

6. Stretch channels: still poorly explored

In the cardiovascular system there are several potassium currents that originate from diffrent channels, with different structures [Escande and Standen 1993; Spooner and Brown 1994; Morad et al. 1996] (Figure 2.4, Table 2. 2). (1) There are three main voltage-dependent potassium currents. The transient outward potassium current, I_{to}, which occurs at the beginning of the action potential and is one of the main determinant of its duration; when I_{to} is less active the action potential duration is increased (this current is one of the major determinant of the adaptaion of the myocardium to mechanical overload). The two I_K currents (one is rapid, I_{Kr}, the other is slow, I_{Ks}) are outward delayed rectifier currents, occur latter, and are principally responsible for the repolarization process. (2) The voltage-insensitive currents include I_{K1}, which is an inward rectifier background current occurring during the rest period and which slightly corrects the resting potential, and two ligand-activated currents, one that is activated by acetylcholine (in the conduction system) and another that is inactivated by ATP (during ischemia).

Ion channels and ion currents

Channels are holes in the membranes, but holes whose gating is regulated (Figure 2. 5, Table 2. 2). The ionic movement is indeed commanded both by the ionic gradient and the degree of opening of the channel. Ion channels are complex proteins encoded by multiple genes that have been already cloned.

Voltage-gated plasma-membrane cation channels. These form a protein family that have a common motif, the voltage sensor, and that is subdivided into two subgroups: the calcium and sodium channels and the voltage-sensitive potassium channels [reviewed in Catterall 1994; Spooner and Brown 1994; Morad et al. 1996]. These proteins are composed of several subunits: sodium and calcium channels are made from one principal and several auxiliary subunits (α, $\beta1$, MW 260, 38 kd, and $\beta2$ for the sodium channel; $\alpha1$, $\alpha2$, β, γ and δ, MW 175, 143, 54, 30 and 27 kd, for the L type calcium channel); voltage-gated (also called Shaker-type) potassium channels are slightly different and have four principal and equivalent subunits and no auxiliary subunits.

The primary structure of the principal subunit of the sodium or calcium channels and that of the principal subunits of the potassium channels is based on the same domain (Figure2. 7). Structural studies have revealed strong analogies between the different domains from which the ion channels are made. In sodium and calcium channels the main subunit consists of four homologous transmembrane domains that surround the central pore. Each of the four domains contains six transmembrane hydrophobic α-helices called S1-S6. In the voltage-gated potassium channels these domains are very similar to those of the Na and Ca channels. Nevertheless, each domain is a separate peptide encoded by a separate gene and the functional subunit of the channel is in fact a heterotetramer (Escande and Standen 1993; Morad et al. 1996). In other words, each potassium channel is composed of four quarters of a sodium channel, and the possibility of potassium channel subunits assembling into heteromultimeric channels provides a structural basis for the generation of a rich variety of functioning channel proteins.

The pore-forming region of the voltage-sensitive channels is formed by four pairs of transmembrane helices (S5 and S6) and the corresponding connecting sequence, H5 (Fig. 2. 5). The S4 transmembrane segment is responsible for the activation of the channel and acts as a voltage-sensor - that is a protein fragment whose spatial structure is sensitive to changes in voltage and is therefore able to transmit a cellular message to the whole protein. The S4 fragment is helicoidal and is made from repeated groups of three amino acids composed by a positively charged amino acid followed by two hydrophobic residues (residue is commonly used as a synonymous of amino acid). For example, neutralization of several positively charged residues can be obtained by mutagenesis. It results in substantial shifts of voltage-dependence. Inactivation is a process that differs from one type of channel to another. From a structural point of view, the intracellular loop connecting domain III to domain IV forms a hinged lid that can alternatively occlude the intracellular mouth of the pore. In potassium channels the structural basis of inactivation is very similar, but the lid is more like a ball and chain, and the portion of the peptide that is responsible for the occlusion of the pore is located at the amino terminal of the peptide.

Phosphorylation of the calcium channels activates the gating of the channel and by so doing enhances the inward calcium current and the duration of the action potential. Sodium channels are also phosphorylatable by cAMP: phosphorylation has a different effect depending on the membrane potential. The genes encoding the a-subunit of the Na and Ca channel are known: a mutation on the Na channel subunit a is responsible for one of the forms of the long QT syndrome (*LQT3*) (see Chapter 4 Genetics for nongeneticians).

The channels responsible for I_{kur} and I_{to} are heterotetramers. I_{ks} is another type of K channel responsible for delayed rectification and a major determinant of the duration of the action potential. Mutation on the corresponding channel (also called *minK*) can also cause congenital long QTsyndrome.

Voltage-insensitive channels. The inward rectifier background channel, responsible for I_{k1}, is different from the voltage-dependent K channels and composed only of two transmembrane segments (M1 and M2, linked by H5). M1 and M2 are very like S5 and S6 and form the pore of the inward rectifier. Nevertheless, this channel does not possess the voltage sensor helix S4, and therefore the corresponding channel is insensitive to changes in voltage. The corresponding genes (*Kir 2.1, 2.2, 2.3*) have recently been cloned and expressed [Morad et al. 1996]. The K_{ATP} channel is a heteromultimer consisting of a pore-forming unit formed by 4 molecules of *Kir 6.2*, which is a member of the inwardly rectifying K^+ channel family, surrounded by 4 regulatory subunits, called *SUR1*, which is a sulfonylurea receptor essential for the activation of the K_{ATP} channel by MgADP.

In the calcium-dependent potassium channels, sequence analysis has revealed high-affinity binding sites for calcium. In cyclic nucleotide-gated channels, such as cAMP- or cGMP- (in the vessels) gated channels, gating depends on binding of the ligand on a consensus sequence for binding the cyclic nucleotide that resembles that of the cyclic nucleotide-dependent protein kinases. The acetylcholine nicotinic receptor is a cationic channel that is regulated by acetylcholine and mediates the transduction in the autonomous system at the ganglionic level. It is made up of five subunits that form a channel. Each subunit is made from four transmembrane spanning domains and an intracellular loop between domain 3 and 4 containing an amphipatic helix which interacts with a cytoskeleton-bridging protein. There is much evidence to suggest that domain 2 lines the aqueous ion channel.

Gap-junctions. These are the largest ion channels of the cardiovascular system, ensure the propagation of action potential between myocytes, and are made from polymorphic proteins called *connexins* (CX) [Gros and Jongsma 1996]. 14 CXs have been identified so far in mammalian heart. Each CX is encoded by a single gene, and each gene consists of two exons separated by a large intron of several kb. CXs oligomerizes into homo- or hetero-hexameric channels, which are termed *connexons*, and two connexons, in adjacent cells, align to form a junctional channel, called *gap-junction*, spanning the external membranes of the two cells to be connected. Hence, the gap-junction channel has a structure very similar to that of the voltage-gated channels described above. Nevertheless, the hole is bigger and has 6 connexin instead of 4 domains or subunits. Mammalian cardiocytes are associated with three developmentally regulated CXs, CX43 (which is the major isoform), CX40 (which has the greatest conductance) and CX45. CX37 is specific for the endothelial cells. Several *in vitro* systems have been developed to study the expression of various isoCXs and to evaluate their functionality in terms of voltage-sensitivity of their electrical conductance, and it has been demonstrated that CX45 possesses the highest voltage-sensitivity.

The sinus node. This has a very particular composition in terms of ion channels and receptors. The sodium current is absent, and there are no connexons. There are several K channels and two new currents that are not present in non differentiated myocardium (Table 2. 2) namely I_{CaT}, which is a calcium inward current insensitive to calcium blockers, and I_f, which is a diastolic current responsible for the spontaneous depolarisation of the sinus node core cells. I_f is likely to be the major determinant of the pacemaker activity and is often termed *pacemaker current.* Specific inhibitors of I_f exist and cause bradycardia: I_f is sensitive to β-blockers [Di Francesco 1986; Mangin et al. 1998]. The sinus node ion channels are responsible for the heart rate on an isolated or a freshly transplanted heart. *In vivo* the heart rate is modified by the activity of the ANS and becomes more rapid than the pacemaker because of the predominancy of the vagal tone in human. The sinus node contains more β-adrenergic and more muscarinic receptors than the rest of the atria.

Intracellular ion homeostasis

Calcium homeostasis

Calcium is a major intracellular messenger that plays a role non only in muscles but also in nearly all other cells. In cardiac and vascular smooth muscle, the function of calcium is to transmit the electrical signal to the sarcomere in order to trigger the mechanical event. In all cells, including myocytes, calcium has two origins: the extracellular space and the endoplasmic reticulum. The importance of these two sources varies from one type of muscle to another but also, for a given type of muscle, from one animal species to the other. For example, the fast skeletal muscle of a rabbit is able to contract in a calcium-free medium because all the calcium used for contraction comes from the sarcoplasmic reticulum (SR). On the other hand, in the frog ventricle that possesses very little SR, contraction is triggered only by external calcium. The rat ventricle is close to the skeletal model: nevertheless, external calcium plays a role and the muscle can't contract in a calcium-free medium. The human ventricle nearly equally utilizes both sources of calcium. Such phylogenic differences explain why the biological process of adaptation to mechanical overload is not the same in every species.

Calcium transient. The intracellular concentration of calcium is maintained between 10nM and 10mM. The so-called physiological calcium transient is located between these two limits (Figure 2. 6). The calcium transient is an increase in intracellular calcium concentration that is triggered by a voltage change; it follows the electrical event, precedes contraction, and can be directly measured by using specific fluorescent compounds that bind free calcium, such as aequorine, indo-1 or fura. Figure 2. 6a shows the time-course of the events with calcium increase preceding contraction. It also shows evidence of a direct relationship both between the amount of external calcium present into the medium and the intracellular calcium concentration $[Ca]_i$ and between $[Ca]_i$ and the increase in force. Most of the inotropic drugs acts through an increase in $[Ca]_i$.

Figure 2. 6b shows simultaneously the effects of a variation in calcium concentration on force in a membrane-free (skinned) preparation and also on actomyosin ATPase activity; the two curves superimpose. The upper limit is imposed by the intracellular concentration of free phosphate, which is around 10mM. Such a concentration is high enough to precipitate calcium as calcium phosphate when the intracellular concentration of free calcium reaches 10mM. Calcium homeostasis is obtained as long as the free $[Ca]_i$ remains below such a threshold. During acute ischemia, the external membrane becomes permeable to calcium, and the intracellular concentration of calcium exceeds the threshold of 10mM. This results in the formation of

A. Calcium transient

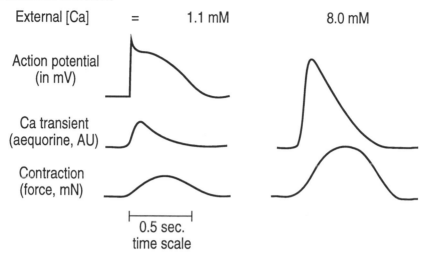

External [Ca]   =   1.1 mM   8.0 mM

Action potential
(in mV)

Ca transient
(aequorine, AU)

Contraction
(force, mN)

0.5 sec.
time scale

B. Threshold for contraction

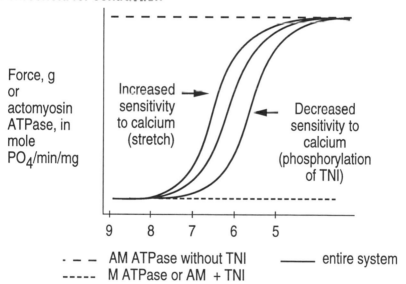

Force, g
or
actomyosin
ATPase, in
mole
PO_4/min/mg

Increased
sensitivity
to calcium
(stretch)

Decreased
sensitivity to
calcium
(phosphorylation
of TNI)

9   8   7   6   5

- – – AM ATPase without TNI   ——— entire system
- - - - M ATPase or AM + TNI

Fig. 2.6. The two components of the calcium transient

calcium phosphate which precipitates as calcifictions around the infarcted zone.

[Ca]$_i$ originates from both the extracellular space and the intracellular stores (Figure 2. 7). Calcium concentration in all cells peaks around 1mM and then binds calciproteins (Figure 2. 8) to activate contraction and metabolism. Consequently, the calcium concentration returns rapidly to low levels, around 0.1mM, owing to active mechanisms located either on the external membrane or on the SR.

Determinants of calcium movement. In any tissue, calcium homeostasis and calcium transient depends on two groups of proteins: those that are in charge of calcium uptake and those which activate release of calcium (Figure 2. 7). The calcium gradient between the cytosol and either the external medium or the extracytosolic compartment or the SR, is around 20,000 nM, which means that calcium does not need energy to enter the cytosol (it is only necessary to gate a channel), whereas calcium release needs directly or indirectly a lot of energy to pull out calcium against the gradient.

The two gates responsible for calcium uptake are calcium channels located either on the sarcolemma (SL), or on the SR: the latter are called *ryanodine receptors*. The Ca channels of SL are voltage-gated in all cells, but, in addition, there are also receptor-operated channels (ROC) in the blood vessels. In the heart, the sinus pacemaker transmits a wave of depolarization through the conduction system to every Ca channels in the cardiocytes. The voltage change gates the channels and allows calcium to enter the cell and triggers contraction both directly and through the ryanodine receptors (Ca-induced Ca-release phenomena) [Fabiato 1981].

The contraction of smooth muscle cells in the vessels depends on various mediators (see further) including norepinephrine, endothelin and angio II. Most of the corresponding receptors, such as adrenergic receptors,

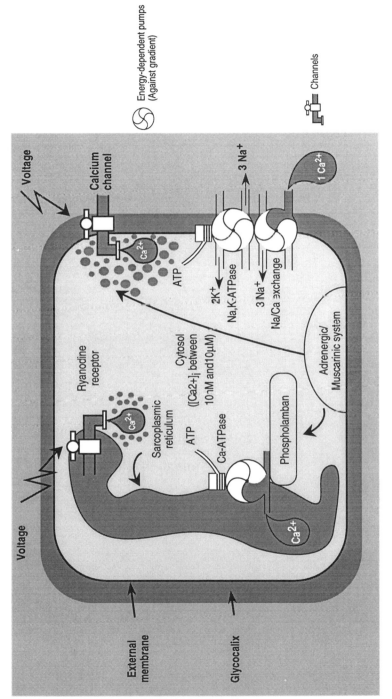

Fig. 2.7. Main determinants of the intracellular calcium homeostasis

A. E-F Hand structure
of a calcium binding site

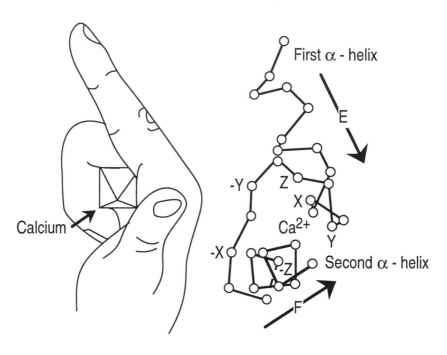

B. Octaedric structure of
calcium coordination sites

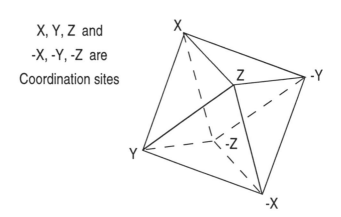

Fig. 2.8. Calciproteins [redrawn from Kretsinger and Barry, 1975]

are on the terminal ends of the nerves and exist only on the cells located at the periphery of the vascular wall. In these cells contraction is triggered by the ROC and is then propagated to voltage-operated Ca channels of other cells that are located more deeply in the vascular wall. Vascular ryanodine receptors are also activated by various mediators and are sensitive to IP3.

Ca^{2+} release also depends on both SL and SR. At the level of the SL, there are two mechanisms (Figure 2. 10): the Na^+/Ca^{2+} exchange that is able to both release and take up calcium but is usually working as a Ca^{2+} release system (see also Figure 2. 7), and the plasma membrane Ca^{2+} ATPase (PMCA). The exchanger indirectly uses the energy of the Na^+, K^+-ATPase, the sodium pump, since it needs a low internal sodium concentration to be allowed to do its job. Digitalis, by blocking the Na^+, K^+-ATPase, increases the calcium concentration through the Na^+/Ca^{2+} exchanger. PMCA is rather poorly active in the heart, but the smooth muscle isoform is very active. Calcium uptake from the SR depends on a Ca^{2+}ATPase that is, in both the smooth and the cardiac muscles, regulated by phospholamban, a cAMP dependent phosphoprotein.

Plasma membrane calcium-regulating proteins. In most of mammalians, the Ca inward current that is controlled by the Ca channel is more likely to trigger the release of calcium from SR than to significatively enhance $[Ca]_i$ (see above and Fig. 2. 7). Exchangers and cotransporters are membrane proteins that have evolved to fulfil general functions such as the maintenance of calcium homeostasis and pH. They have a similar structure and span the membrane about 12 times (instead of 7 for the R7G). The most important components of this family in the cardiovascular system are, for the moment, the Na^+/Ca^{2+} exchanger and the Na^+/H^+ exchangers (or antiporters).

The Na^+/Ca^{2+} exchanger is highly expressed in the myocardium where it is the major pathway for the extrusion of calcium out of the cell

[Reithmeier 1994; Morad et al. 1996]. The exchanger is electrogenic, creates a current (Fig. 2. 7) and exchanges one calcium for 3 sodiums. It can function in the 2 directions: nevertheless, because of the normal stoichiometry of the two cations, it normally releases calcium out of the cell and acts as a major determinant of both diastole and vasodilation, and the current is predominantly an ourward current. The protein (MW 120 Kd) has 970 amino acids that are arranged into 11 putative transmembrane segments with a large cytosolic domain located between segments 5 and 6 [Morad et al. 1996]. Such a cytosolic domain contains a calmodulin-binding site and regulatory elements sensitive to a specific inhibitory peptide. In humans, the protein is encoded by one gene that contains 6 central exons encoding the cytosolic loop and that, by alternative splicing, can make 32 different transcripts specific for different tissues (cardiac, renal, and brain isoforms have been identified). The cardiac specific isoform is called NCX1. NCX2, the brain isoform, is present in the heart in very low amount.

Recent studies have demonstrated the existence of a functionally active calmodulin-dependent plasma membrane calcium ATPase that may play a major role in releasing calcium both in the heart and in the smooth muscle of the vessels. This ATPase is encoded by four different genes, each alternatively spliced at several different positions.

Sarcoplasmic reticulum (SR). Both in the heart and vascular smooth muscle cells, the sarcoplasmic reticulum, SR, consists of tubules (10 to 50 nm in diameter) that anastomose, divide in all directions, and form a lacelike network that wraps around myofibrils and spreads across the Z-line discs. A specialized part of the SR is called *junctional* and lies in proximity to the T tubules of the plasma membrane and forms triads. In skeletal muscle, triads are structures connected one to each other through a protein called *foot*. In the heart the connection between SR and SL is mostly functional. The main function of the SR is to store and release calcium and to couple contraction

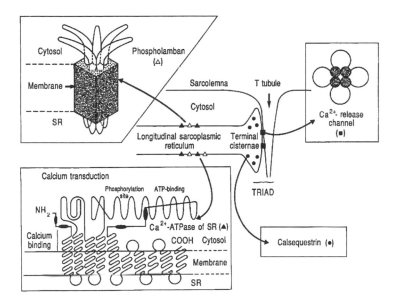

Fig. 2.9. Proteins of the sarcoplasmic reticulum. Middle: triad, periphery: proteins [from Swynguedauw 1990, with permission].

106

A. Calcium-induced calcium-release in the heart

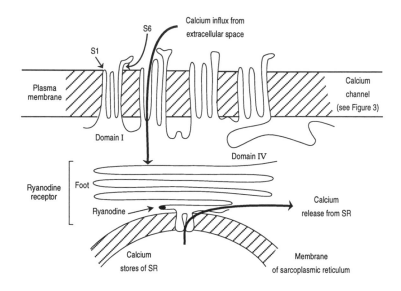

B. IP3-induced calcium-release in the vessels

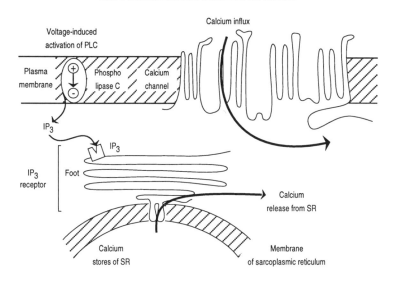

Fig. 2.10 Structural basis for the cardiac calcium-induced calcium release (A) and the vascular IP3-induced calcium-release (B) in the SR.

with electrical activity. Figure 2. 9. shows the main proteins that play a functional role in the SR: (1) uptake of calcium is against the gradient, needs energy and is controlled by a Ca-ATPase; (2) calcium storage depends on a calciprotein (see below), calsequestrine, which binds a considerable amount of calcium per mole (about 40); and (3) calcium release differs from one type of muscle to another and depends upon rather complex calcium channels, termed *ryanodine receptor* in the heart, and *IP3 receptor* in the vessels. Ryanodine and IP3 receptor are very homologous proteins but are encoded by different genes.

The Ca-ATPase was first isolated from fast skeletal muscle, where it is the most abundant. The density of the Ca ATPase in SR is approximately 6,000 higher than that of the Ca channels of SL. The enzyme is able to transport two calcium molecules per molecule of ATP hydrolyzed and belongs to the P-type class of ATPases (Table 2. 1). The model shown in Figure 2. 10. includes 10 helical hydrophobic segments, M1-10 (2 high affinity calcium binding sites have been identified in a channel created by M4, 5, 6 and 8) connected to 3 cytosolic hydrophilic loops, which contain both the ATP binding site and the phosphorylation site. Several isoforms are now well-characterized (the cardiac isoform is termed SERCA 2a, MW 105-115 kD). These enzymes are encoded by at least 3 genes, all of which may be alternatively spliced to generate different protein isoforms.

The cardiac and vascular isoforms have the particularity to be regulated by a protein, acting as a cofactor, phospholamban that is present in a molar ratio of 1:1 (and that does not exist into the skeletal muscle). Phospholamban is a pentamer made up of 5 subunits (MW 6,000 D) that form a sort of tunnel. Each subunit is phosphorylatable and posses 2 different phosphorylation sites that correspond to 2 different protein kinases, one that is the cAMP-dependent protein kinase protein kinase C and the other that is calmodulin-dependent. The phosphorylation of phospholamban induces transconformational changes of the calcium ATPase whose pumping ability is, in turn, activated. The increased rate of relaxation (also called the *lusinotropic effect*) that is observed after β-agonist stimulation is due to an enhanced uptake of calcium by SR, which, in turn, corresponds to the phosphorylation of phospholamban by cAMP and the activation of the calcium ATPase.

The calcium release from SR is directly or indirectly voltage-dependent, and the mechanism of the calcium release from SR varies from one muscle to the other. In the fast skeletal muscle the release depends on a spanning protein that directly transmits the voltage change to the calcium channel of the SR. In the heart (Figure 2. 10) the release is autocatalytic and triggered by the calcium inward current which transmits the signal to the ryanodine receptor (ryanodine is a synthetic marker that does not exist *in vivo*). In the vessels the release is commanded by voltage-dependent IP3 production from the phosphoinositol cycle (Figure 2. 10) and the signal, (IP3), acts on an IP3 receptor, which is also the calcium channel of SR.

In the SR, there are at least 3 calcium-release channels isoforms [Coronado et al. 1994] (Figure 2. 10). These channels are different from the plasma membrane dihydropyridine-sensitive calcium channels described above. The protein is a tetramer and comprises 4 subunits (MW around 500 kD) that forms a channel. Each subunit is composed by 4 hydrophobic transmembrane segments (called M1, 2, 3, and 4) that anchor this bulky protein to the SR membrane and a hydrophilic cytoplasmic domain termed foot.

Membrane depolarization, as neurotransmitters or hormones, evokes a release of calcium from SR stores through these calcium channels. Nevertheless, from a pure physiological point of view, the important point is that the calcium release from SR is not permanent. The release is pulsatory and triggered by voltage changes.

Calciproteins. Phospholipids or DNA bind divalent cations. Nevertheless, because of the high intracellular Mg^{2+} concentration (1 mM), proteins are the only molecules that bind calcium with a pKd (Ca) of 5 to 7. Calcium-binding proteins, or calciproteins, have either a high capacity and low affinity for Ca^{2+} or low capacity but high affinity. Calcium modifies their properties and/or stability. Finally, both the function and interactions of the protein depend on calcium binding.

It has been demonstrated that a large number of calciproteins possess one or several calcium binding sites that have a common consensus amino acid sequence, termed the *E-F hand structure* (Figure 2. 8), and include 2 turns of α-helix, a 12-residue loop containing 6 calcium-coordinating ligands that maintain calcium in a pocket, and again 2 turns of α-helix. A model has been proposed, based on the structure of parvalbumin, a calciprotein with very high affinity for calcium. It is generally admitted that the affinity for calcium of a given binding site is higher when the structure is close to the model [Kretsinger and Barry 1975].

Calciproteins include parvalbumin (a Ca^{2+} transporter in certain muscles), troponin C, the nonphosphorylated myosin light chain that has incomplete E-F hand regions, suggesting that calcium affinity is low, calsequestrin, and, very likely, the Ca-ATPase of SR. Calmodulin has 4 homologous divalent cationic binding sites and is active as (3 Ca^{2+}-1 Mg^{2+}). It is the cofactor of a large number of enzymes, including myosin light chain kinase (predominant in the vessels), phosphodiesterase, adenylate cyclase, glycogen synthetase and phosphorylase, phospholamban, and the protein responsible for microtubular disassembly.

The E-F hand structure is not the only structure able to bind calcium. Other consensus structures for a calcium-binding site have been reported - for example that found in calcimedin, endonexin, calelectrin, calpactin and lipocortin and which consists of 17 aminoacids that form a loop followed by an α-helix.

The sodium/potassium homeostasis

Na^+, K^+-ATPase, the so-called sodium pump, is directly responsible for intracellular sodium and potassium homeostasis and indirectly responsible for that of calcium, because the enzyme is coupled with the Na^+/Ca^{2+} exchange. Hydrolysis of one molecule of ATP permits the release of 3 Na^+ ions and the uptake of 2 K^+ ions, each against the electrochemical gradients. The enzyme creates a sodium gradient which is used by the cell to drive numerous transport process, including the Na^+/Ca^{2+} exchange and the Na^+/H^+ exchange. As a consequence, the sodium pump is electrogenic and takes part in the repolarization of the membrane with each excitation-contraction cycle. This ATPase belongs to the P-type class of ATPases, which also includes the plasma membrane calcium ATPase and the calcium ATPase of the SR (Table 2. 2). These enzymes share a similar catalytic cycle that involves a phosphorylated protein intermediate. An important notion is that the enzyme consumes approximately 20% of the ATP at rest in the whole organism, which renders Na^+/K^+ homeostasis an extremely expensive procedure and alterations of the activity of this pump a sensitive tool to oxygene-deprivation.

Digitalis and related compounds (ouabain) bind specifically to Na^+, K^+-ATPase. Inhibition of the enzyme by cardiac glycosides provokes an increase in intracellular sodium and subsequently of calcium via the Na^+/Ca^{2+} exchange. This increase in calcium will, in turn, cause the inotropic effect (the mechanism of which is not as simple since the inotropic effect is only systolic, and not diastolic, as expected).

The sodium pump is a dimer comprising one α-subunit (MW 112 kd) carrying all the known receptor sites of the enzyme and one glycosylated β-subunit, which is indispensable for the activity [Lingrel 1994]. The most up-to-date working model of membrane topology includes ten transmembrane domains (called H1... H10), divided into 2 groups - a group of 4 on the N-terminal side and a group of 6 on the C-terminal side. Multiple extracellular and transmembrane regions are involved in determining ouabain sensitivity; this area of research is still in process. Ouabain binds on the external side, and the hydrolytic site is located on the intracellular side.

Both subunits are polymorphic. Three isoforms of the α-subunits are presently known. In the rat $\alpha 1$ is an ubiquitous form present in every tissues and has a low affinity to ouabain and high affinity for sodium; $\alpha 2$ has a high affinity both for ouabain (1,000-fold higher than $\alpha 1$) and for sodium and is found in only a few organs such as the ventricles and the aorta and $\alpha 3$ which embryonic and posses the same high affinity as $\alpha 2$ for ouabain, but has a low affinity for sodium. In humans $\alpha 1$ is different and has a very high affinity for ouabain, and $\alpha 3$ is not specific for embryo and is found during adulthood. Such species differences in normal conditions may explain the species differences observed in cardiac hypertrophy. These 3 isoforms are encoded by three different genes. In the heart, the enzyme has both a low and a high affinity site for ouabain, the first being roughly responsible for toxicity, and the second for inotropic effect. These sites correspond to the α-subunits isoforms, which provide a structural basis for searching for new inotropes with less toxicity. The 3 isoforms are encoded by 3 different isogenes that are both developmentally and hormonally regulated.

Mechanisms to maintain intracellular pH

Cells possess an intrinsec buffering capacity due to the intracellular proteins, phosphates, and above all the CO_2/HCO_3^- content. In addition, the cell can release H^+ when their production exceeds the buffering capacity of the cell. Three mechanisms can play this role, including the passive release of lactic acid, the Na^+/H^+ exchanger (or antiport), and the Na^+-HCO_3 symporter. The Na^+/H^+ exchanger uses the electrochemical gradient as a source of energy to release one proton and to take up in exchange one sodium molecule. The exchanger does not work when the pH is too alkaline and is above 7.3. It is specifically inhibited by amiloride. There are at least 4 isoforms (NHE-1, MW 110KDa, is the cardiac isoform), and the general structure of the antiporter includes 12 transmembrane segments, several phosphorylation sites, a cytoplasmic domain that controls H^+-sensing and a C-terminal cytosolic loop. The antiporter plays a major physiopathologic role during ischemia-reperfusion.

Vascular cell membrane proteins

Vascular contraction is tonic, as compared to myocardial contraction, and is frequently maintained for a long period of time. In parallel, membrane resting and action potential are different since the resting potential in smooth muscle is - 40 to - 55 mV instead of - 80 mV in the heart. The external membrane lacks sodium channels, and the inward current is carried by voltage-dependent and receptor-operated L-type (sensitive to calcium blockers) calcium channels (Table 2. 3) [Tedgui et Levy 1994; Hathaway et al. 1991]. Several K^+ channels have been identified as a major target for vasodilators, including calcium-activated K^+ channel, ATP-sensitive K^+ channel and delayed rectifier potassium channel. Stretch activates cation channels and may depolarize the cell. The smooth muscle SR plays a major role since blocking calcium release from SR by ryanodine stops smooth muscle contraction. Smooth muscle has a specific Ca ATPase isoform and also possesses an active phospholamban that is able to control calcium uptake and produces relaxation exactly as in the heart.

R7-G receptors are present, especially the $\alpha 1$ and $\beta 2$-adrenergic, M3 and M2 muscarinic, angiotensine II, serotonin receptors. These receptors are coupled to several G proteins, including Gs and Gp. Coupling operates through cAMP but also cGMP and the PI cycle. As explained below, most

Table 2. 3. Vascular cell membrane proteins

	Heart	Smooth muscle
Sarcoplasmic Reticulum		
Ca^{2+} ATPase isoforms	cardiac	smooth
Phospholamban	+	+
Ca^{2+} channel of SR	Ca induced	IP3 induced
Ionic Channels		
Na channel	+	0
Ca^{2+} channels	L, T-type	L,T-type like
K^+ channels	I_{to}, I_K, I_{K1}	I_K ? ?
	ACh, ATP	ATP
	Ca-induced	Ca-induced
Na^+, K^+ ATPase subunit α	$\alpha 1, \alpha 2$	$\alpha 1, \alpha 2$
Na^+/Ca^{2+} exchange	+	+
Na^+/H^+ exchange	Specific isoforms	Specific isoforms ?
Connexins subtype	CX 43	CX 43
Receptors		
Adrenergic	$\beta 1, \beta 2, \alpha 1$	$\beta 2, \alpha 1, \alpha 2$
Muscarinic	M2	M3, M2
Angio II	Rare	AT1, AT 2

of the vasoconstricting agents that activate the PI cycle, including angio II, rapidly trigger contraction through the liberation of IP3 and consequently the release of calcium from SR. A second step, which proceeds more slowly, follows and is the diacylglyderol-induced activation of protein kinase C and the corresponding phosphorylations.

SARCOMERE STRUCTURE AND CONTRACTILITY. CYTOSKELETON

Systolic ejection is the ultimate goal of myocardial function and results from the harmonious and simultaneous cyclic contraction of cardiac myocytes. Relaxation of the same cells allows the myocardial filling procedure. In the vessels, contraction is not rhythmic, and relaxation is the way by which the vascular tone is maintained and numerous regulatory peptides regulate this process. In both cardiac and vascular muscles contraction is triggered by the electrical events, the intracellular messenger is calcium, but the origin of the calcium varies according to the species and the type of muscle. Contraction itself results from the sliding of two groups of proteins, called *contractile proteins.*

The sliding process is regulated at the level of the thin filament in the heart (through troponin) and at that of the thick filament in the vessels (through the phosphorylated light chain of myosin). Recently, it has been proposed that the cytoskeleton - that is the cellular net work that maintains the internal structure of the cell - may play an important role during the contractile cycle as it imposes a resistive intracellular load on sarcomere shortening and, formed in excess, impedes sarcomere motion [Tsutsui et al. 1993].

Smooth muscle is not only smooth - that is apparently disorganized as compared to myocardium, which is striated that is highly and geometrically organized - but also the structure of the sarcomere is different, and smooth muscle contractile protein structures and genes differ both from the myocardium and fast skeletal muscles in such a way that antibodies

115

raised against smooth muscle proteins do not cross-react with those raised against striated muscle.

Cardiac sarcomere

Electron micrographs of cardiac fibers show a striated appearance made up of regular alternating dark and light bands (A and I-bands; Figure 2. 11) [Swynghedauw 1986]. In the centre of the A-band is an H-zone and an M-line. The sarcomere is the basic contractile unit - that is the smallest component of the muscle to shorten. It is delimited by the two Z lines. At higher magnification, the sarcomere shows interpenetration of thick (1.5 mm long) and thin filaments (I mm long, start at the Z line). A cross-section at this point shows that each thick filament is surrounded by 6 thin filaments. Thick and thin filaments are interconnected through the myosin bridges projecting from the thick filaments.

Thick filament proteins
The thick filament contains 400 molecules of myosin (MW 500 kD), which is a fibrous protein composed of 2 heavy chains (MW 200 kD) and 2 pairs of light chains (one is phosphorylated, the other is called alkali). Myosin plays an important role in the mechanical events involved in muscle contraction. The structure of the thick filament is bipolar and the myosin molecules are arranged in an antiparallel manner. Myosin bridges are uniformly spaced every 14.3 nm (Figure 2. 11), forming a helix with a coil of 43 nm.

The myosin molecule is made of a long helicoidal rod fragment that contributes to the formation of the filament itself and a head that is the bridge connecting the 2 filaments to each other. The head, also called S1, possesses the sites both for the ATPase activity of the molecule and the binding of actin. There are 2 heads per myosin molecule, and consequently

116

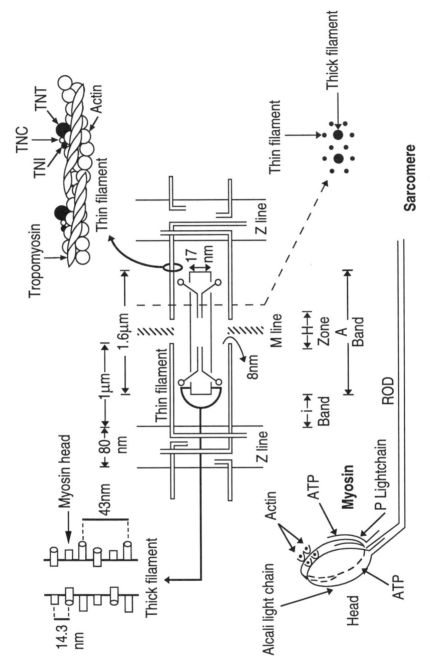

Fig. 2.11 Structure of the striated muscle sarcomere. Middle: structure of a sarcomere, upper right: thin filaments, lower: myosin [from Swynghedauw 1990, with permission].

each molecule of myosin can hydrolyzes 2 molecules of ATP. The active site of the myosin ATPase is located on the myosin heavy chains and the main activator of the enzymatic activity is actin. Cardiac myosin heavy chain isoforms in man and in rat are the products of two highly homologous genes with 40 exons. Theses genes are called α and β, and are located in a head-to-tail arrangement about 4.2 kb apart on chromosome 14. In rat, these two different cardiac myosin heavy chains interact to produce 3 isomyosins, called V_1, V_2, and V_3, which are $\alpha\alpha$, $\alpha\beta$, and $\beta\beta$ myosin heavy chain isoforms, respectively. The cardiac myosin heavy chains are developmentally and tissue regulated, and distinct patterns are observed in ventricles and atria of the same species, as well as in human and rat ventricles. This is, however, always a predominancy of $\alpha\alpha$ in the atria of all species, including humans, and in the rat ventricle. The specific ATPase activity of the α myosin heavy chain isoform is 3 to 4 times higher than that of β and correlates with the maximum shortening velocity of an unloaded cardiac or smooth muscle. The human ventricle has a slower shortening velocity when compared to the rat ventricle and has a higher content of the $\beta\beta$ myosin heavy chain isoforms (in contrast rat ventricle myosin heavy chains are entirely $\alpha\alpha$) [Swynghedauw 1986].

Cardiac myosin light chain isoforms are also heterogeneous. They belong to a monogenic family and are encoded differentially by a process of alternative splicing. Phosphorylated and non phosphorylated light chains are different in the ventricles and in the atria. The nonphosphorylatable atrial light chain is also skeletal embryonic and the corresponding gene is located on chromosome 11. The same light chain in the ventricle is also the slow skeletal muscle light chain, and the gene is on chromosome 9 (in mice).

Thin filament proteins

The thin filaments consist of 2 globular chains of actin 4 nm in diameter twisted into a double helix which contains 13.5 actin molecules per turn

(Figure 2. 11). A coiled-coiled and coiled dimer of tropomyosin occupies the actin-actin cleft. Every 385 nm there is a regulatory complex which is composed of the 3 different troponins, TN, subtypes called TNI, TNC and TNT. The TN complex does not interact directly with myosin: it does so through tropomyosin and actin.

Actin (MW 41,785) isoforms are numerous and encoded by different genes that are located on different chromosomes, and nearly 60 of them, including pseudogenes, have been reported. The striated muscle actin isoforms are a-skeletal (on chromosome 3) and a-cardiac (on chromosome 17) actins which are highly homologous proteins. Both are expressed into the heart. Cardiac TNC and TNI are specific for the myocardium and are encoded by separate genes that are also different from the genes coding for the fast skeletal muscle isoforms. Cardiac TNC (MW 18,459) binds calcium and, by so doing, activates contraction, and this is the last step in excitation-contraction coupling. Nevertheless it has only 3 calcium binding sites, instead of 4 in the skeletal TNC (MW 17,965). Cardiac TNI (MW 23,550) inhibits contraction and is slightly longer than the fast skeletal isoform (MW 20,864). Cardiac TNI is unique because it contains an amino acid that can be phosphorylated by cAMP through a protein kinase C.

Troponin T links TNC and TNI to tropomyosin, and is extremely polymorphic in the heart and the various isoforms are developmentally regulated. TNT (MW 38,000) isoforms are encoded by alternative splicing by the same gene which covers 18 exons. Tropomyosin is a dimer forming a supercoiled double helix 4 nm long that sits in the 2 grooves formed by the twisting of 7 molecules of actin. The actin : tropomyosin stoichiometry is maintained by tropomodulin, which is localized within the region of actin filament pointed ends. Isotropomyosins are homo or heterodimers encoded by 2 different genes α and β, that are, in turn, able to encode by alternative splicing several isoforms.

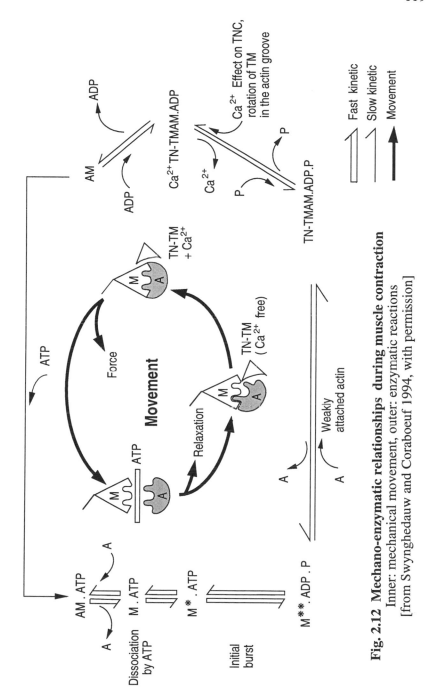

Fig. 2.12 Mechano-enzymatic relationships during muscle contraction
Inner: mechanical movement, outer: enzymatic reactions
[from Swynghedauw and Coraboeuf 1994, with permission]

Contraction movement

When a muscle shortens, the filaments can slide by around 1,000 nm in each sarcomere. Thus the myosin heads cannot remain attached to the same actin monomer but have to be repeatedly attached to and detached from the thin filament of actin. Consequently, shortening could be driven by a preferential attachment of the heads of myosin to upstream actin molecules. Such an attachment stretches the elasticity of the myosin cross-bridges and generates tension. Once the filament has been carried downstream after filament sliding, the myosin head detaches. Contraction is due to the relative sliding of thin and thick filaments due to the movement of the myosin head. Figure 2. 12 summarizes the different steps of contraction in the heart. An important point of this scheme is the dual role of ATP, which is not only the source of energy, as everybody knows, but also the most basic determinant of relaxation. The outer circle shows the enzymatic reaction, and the inner circle is a scheme of the accompanying mechanical movement (M: myosin head; A: actin; TN-TM: troponin-tropomyosin complex). From left to right: (1) relaxation, which is characterized by an inhibition (or a weakening) of the actin-myosin link due to the high concentrations of ATP (the ATPase is no longer active whereas both the mitochondrial and anaerobic synthesis are continue); (2) the initial burst is the first extremely rapid phase of the ATPase reaction: during this step ATP binds to myosin, whose spatial structure changes, it is then hydrolyzed to produce mechanical energy; (3) simultaneously, due to the decrease in ATP concentration, actin binds to myosin, and consequently the tropomyosin-troponin complex is indirectly connected to myosin; the actin-myosin link is still weak because the intracellular calcium concentration is low and TNI hinders the interaction between the two proteins; (4) the increase in the intracellular calcium concentration enhances the affinity of TNC for TNI and instigates a steric and stoichiometric displacement of tropomyosin, which leaves the actin grooves and allows the actin-myosin relationships to be reinforced; actin can then activate the myosin ATPase, the ATP hydrolysis is completed, and the hydrolytic products are released.

Relationships with physiological properties

The tension/length curve is steeper in the heart than in the striated muscle (Figure 2. 13). On a cardiac or skeletal fiber, the length is initial length, or preload, and is a bell-shaped curve, and the top of the bell corresponds to the point where there is a maximum number of actin/myosin bridges formed. Tension in Figure 2. 13, is active tension, and when the tension/length curve is drawn using membrane-free (skinned fibers) samples, it is possible to add ATP and measure ATPase at various lengths. It has been shown that the ATPase/length curve has the same bell-shaped appearance as the curve obtained with fresh tissue. *In vivo* the length corresponds to the end-diastolic volume and active tension to the pressure developed.

The velocity/after-load curve is drawn at a constant preload (or initial length), and Vmax is the initial shortening velocity for unloaded muscle. Vmax depends on the maximum myosin ATPase activity which, in turn, is determined by the genetic characteristics of the molecule, the number of actin molecules bound to myosin (that is, the load), and also, with some restrictions, the intracellular calcium concentration. The myosin ATPase enzymatic site is located on the heads of the heavy chains, and, from a genetic point of view, depend on the isoform that is present. In phylogeny, in various muscles from different animal species, myosin ATPase, the biochemical parameter, is positively correlated with Vmax, the physiological parameter. Such a phylogenetic relationships is also found in cardiac diseases.

122

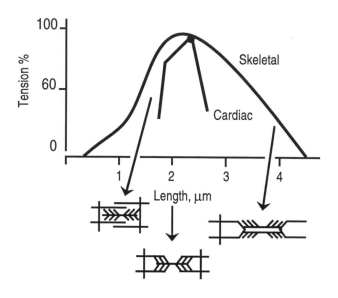

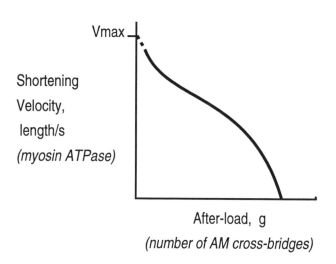

Fig. 2.13 Physiological-molecular correspondences of contractility.
Upper: active tension/length curve, lower: velocity/length curve.

Smooth muscle sarcomere

Smooth muscle cells are located in the media of the arterial wall. The vascular smooth muscle sarcomere is arranged differently (Figure 2. 14). As opposed to striated muscle (Table 2.4), the structure of the smooth muscle sarcomere is unipolar and myosin molecules are parallel.

Table 2. 4. Smooth muscle sarcomere.

	Heart	Smooth muscle
Contraction.		
Type	Phasic	Tonic
Refractory period	⊢	0
Contractile proteins.		
Myosin heavy chains	α and β	1 and 2
P MLC	2_V and 2_A	20kD, 2 isoforms
Alkali MLC	1_V and 1_A	17kD, 2 isoforms
Actin	α-card/skel	α-smooth
Tropomyosin	$\alpha2$-, β-cardiac	$\alpha3$-, β-smooth
Troponins C and I	cardiac specific	no TN
Troponin T	several isoforms	no TN
M LC Kinase activity	poor	important
Calponin	0	+
Caldesmon	0	+

In addition, the smooth muscle contains less myosin and more actin per g of tissue than does the cardiac tissue (the actin/myosin ratio is indeed 4 in the striated muscle and 35 in the arterial smooth muscle), which gives

124

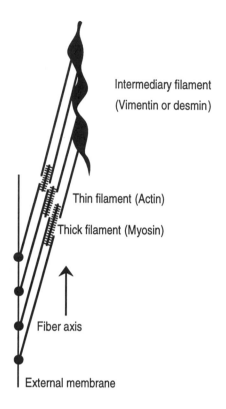

Intermediary filament
(Vimentin or desmin)

Thin filament (Actin)

Thick filament (Myosin)

Fiber axis

External membrane

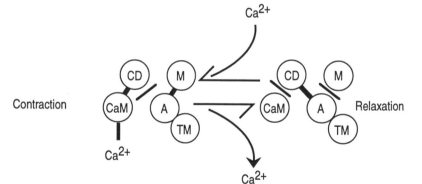

Fig. 2.14. Structure of the smooth muscle.
Upper: sarcomere, lower: regulation of contraction

the sarcomere a very particular shape (Fig. 2. 14). Smooth muscle isoactins are β and γ isoforms and are different from the striated muscle isoforms. Troponin is absent from smooth muscle, but tropomyosin is present (Table 2. 4). Smooth muscle contains only 30% of the myosin found in myocardium. Nevertheless, they develop the same range of force because the force produced per myosin head is 3-fold higher in smooth muscle than in striated muscles. In addition, the smooth muscle myosin is much more efficient than the striated muscle and uses less ATP per cross-bridge. Myosin subunits of the smooth muscle are also polymorphic, but the physiological significance of this polymorphism has not yet been explored in detail. The contractile activity of the smooth muscle is also regulated by calcium. Nevertheless, the mechanism of the regulation is different since there is no troponin in the smooth muscle.

In smooth muscle the regulation of contraction depends on the state of phosphorylation of the phosphorylatable myosin light chain. Phosphorylation of this subunit is the signal that increases the rate constant of the rate-limiting step in the actomyosin ATPase cycle, activates the cycling of the cross-bridges, and initiates the mechanical event. The light chains are phosphorylated by a specific kinase (MW 160 kD), which is activated by calcium through calmodulin (CaM). Myosin light chain phosphorylation is correlated both with the intracellular calcium concentration and the velocity of muscle shortening. The affinity of the myosin light chain kinase for CaM decreases when the kinase is itself phosphorylated by protein kinase C. Such a mechanism explains the vasodilatory effects of adrenergic agonists. A characteristic feature of smooth muscle is that during the contraction cycle, muscle tension increases more slowly than shortening and is maintained at a reduced ATP consumption while the calcium concentration decreases. This so-called latch state reflects a very specific regulation of contraction and may be related to other proteins. caldesmon (CD) (Figure 2. 14), is one of these, it is a phosphorylatable calmodulin-dependent protein that competes with myosin on actin. When calcium binds CaM, caldesmon can no longer bind actin and contraction occurs.

To summarize, the cardiac smooth muscle is made up of specific contractile proteins different from those of the myocardium. It contains less myosin, and more actin than the striated muscle. The regulation of the smooth muscle contraction is located on the thick filament because smooth muscle does not contain troponin, and involves the cAMP and calcium-dependent phosphorylation of a specific myosin light chain.

Cytoskeleton

In any cell, the cytoskeleton consists in a rather complex network of proteins that maintains the shape of the cell and links the cells one another. The destruction of the cytoskeleton is one of the most crucial determinant of irreversibility after ischaemic myocardial injury [Ganote and Armstrong 1993]. Cytoskeleton is also likely to play an important role to transduce external signals to nucleus during the process of cardiac overload [Rappaport and Samuel 1988] and to maintain internal force [Tsutsui et al. 1993].

The general organization of the cell is assured by an intermediate system of desmin (although vimentin is expressed in early embryos) filaments (10nm diameter), which are arranged as longitudinal intercommunicating fibres running between myofibres from one desmosome to another and connect to mitochondria and nuclei. The transverse system encircles myofibres at the Z bands and connect to the external membrane the extracellular matrix, ECM, at the lateral costamere junctions (Figure 2. 15, Table 2. 5).

The sarcomere structure (see above cardiac sarcomere and below smooth muscle sarcomere) is maintained by a dense and complex network that is related to internal force transmission. Sarcomeres are linked to one another at Z bands (Fig. 2. 11) and to external membrane at fascia adherens and lateral costamere junctions (Fig. 2. 15). The Z band is organized as a region of overlapping tails of thin filaments of actin cross-linked by $\alpha-$ actinin dimers and connected to desmin intermediate filaments by α-crystallin, Z band also includes several actin capping proteins, such as $CapZ_{(36/32)}$, gelsolin, or β-actinin. The longitudinal structure of sarcomere is maintained by a thin elastic component, *titin*, which connects the sarcomere proteins during contractile cycle and may play a crucial role during relaxation. The bundles of thick filaments are maintained by M lines proteins and principally by the C-protein and the M-protein. Mutations on the C-protein creates hypertrophy.

Microtubules cross the cells from the nucleus to subsarcolemmal region [Rappaport and Samuel 1988]. This is a rather thick network, 10 to 30 nm in diameter, due to the polymerization of polymorphic dimeric proteins, called *tubulin*, by kinases, the *microtubules associated kinases* and *Tau (T) factor*. Microtubules are essential components for the cardiac growth during development and cardiac hypertrophy and play a mechanical role as a linker.

The cardiocyte connect to other cardiocytes across the intercalated disk and to the extracellular matrix, ECM, through lateral adherens junctions. The intercalated disk consists in nexus, or gap-junctions, that are formed by the connexons (see above), desmosomes that are composed of a cytoplasmic plaque of attachment proteins and link the intermediate filaments from one cell to another, and adherens junctions of fascia adherens. The *fascia adherens* which is the site of cell-to-cell contact across the intercalated disk, links the sarcomere of adjacent cells and consists of an assembly of attachment proteins including A-CAM (adherens junction specific cell adhesion molecule), plakoglobulin (or α-catenin in other cells), tensin, metavinculin, and vinculin (a molecule shaped like a balloon on a string), which binds to α-actinin and through this intermediary to actin filament.

Table 2. 5. Cardiocyte cytoskeleton [from Ganote and Armstrong 1993; Rappaport and Samuel 1988; Farhadian et al. 1996]. XX means multiple isoforms. MAP: microtubules-associated proteins. A-CAM: Ca dependent cadherin.

Protein	Mass in kDa	Function
INTERCONNECTING FILAMENTS		
Microtubules		
Tubulin	55/53 (XX)	Binds organelles, development
MAP	300	Regulates assembly
Tau factor	60	Activates assembly
Intermediate filaments (10nm diameter)		
Desmin	55	Surrounds myofibrils, links
		nucleus/ SL /mito/desmosomes
PROTEINS OF THE SARCOMERE		
Z disc		
Actin	42 (XX)	Contraction
β-actinin	34 (XX)	Actin-capping
α-actinin	95	Actin cross-linking
CapZ	36 (XX)	Actin-capping
α-Crystallin	20	Desmin binding
M line		
Myosin	500 (XX)	Contraction
M protein	165	Myosin binding
C protein	140	Myosin binding
Creatine kinase	80 (XX)	Energy transduction
Titin	>1,000 (XX)	Elastic, links actin/myosin
		along sarcomere

CELL-TO-CELL CONNECTING PROTEINS

Connexons

Connexins	37 to 45 (XX)	Intercellular channels

Desmosomes (intercalated disks)

Desmoplakin, Plakoglobin, Desmogelin

Proteins of fascia adherens junctions

(A-CAM)	135	Links two adjacent cells across the EC space
Plakoglobulin	83	Binds A-CAM/vinculin play an α-catenin function
Vinculin	117	Links α-catenin/a-actinin
α-actinin	82	Links vinculin/actin

Proteins of lateral adherens junction and basal membrane

Integrin	130 (XX)	Transmembrane protein, links talin/collagen
Talin	213	Links integrin/vinculin
Vinculin	117	Links talin/a-actinin
Dystrophin	400	Links actin/β-dystroglycan
β-dystroglycan	complex	Links dystrophin to basal membrane

The *lateral*, or *costamere, adherens junctions* link the sarcomere to the collagen network, basal membrane, and surface membrane glycoproteins across the lateral external membrane. The attachment proteins are different from that of the fascia adherens and include talin and integrins, which are transmembrane polymorphic proteins, and dystrophin, which is a large subsarcolemmal and transmembrane protein whose mutations cause Duchenne muscular dystrophy. Dystrophin exists in the heart and links the sarcomere to a transmembrane complex, dystroglycane, which itself binds the basal membrane proteins, fibronectine and laminin. Paxillin, another

130

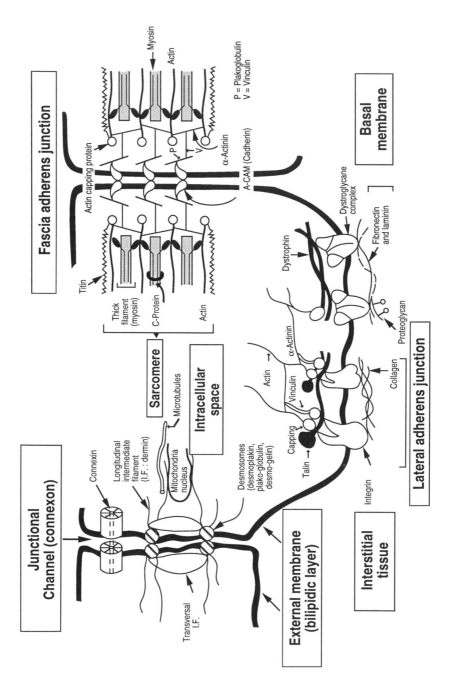

Fig. 2.15 Cardiocyte cytoskeleton

component of costamere junctions, is found in smooth muscles and fibroblasts. The lipid bilayer of external membrane is both stabilized and linked to cytoskeleton by a complex subcortical membrane lattice that is composed by several proteins, including spectrin, ankyrin, filamin, and some specific membrane isoforms of actin.

EXTRACELLULAR MATRIX AND TISSUE COMPLIANCE

Extracellular matrix (ECM)

Cardiac myocytes and capillaries are surrounded by an extensive connective tissue lattice work that is mainly composed of collagen but also contains glycosaminoglycans, elastin and fibronectin. *ECM* is linked to cells across lateral fascia adherens (see above). ECM is certainly much more dynamic than previously believed and is not only a support for myocytes and an extracellular skeleton but also controls the morphology and phenotype of cells, specially during development. Fibronectin is particularly known to affect cell adhesion, migration and cytodifferentiation and is implicated in organogenesis. Three levels of myocardial connective tissue have been described (Figure 2. 16): epimysium envelops the entire cardiac muscle; perimysium associates groups of cells; and endomysium supports and interconnects individual myocytes [Brilla et al. 1990; Weber et al. 1993]. Each myocyte is linked to adjacent cells by struts of collagen of 150 nm diameter, which run perpendicularly to the basement membranes and prevent excessive elongation or shortening of the cardiocytes. They also synchronize myocyte contraction by uniformly disseminating tension so that cells are equally elongated during contraction and store energy during the cardiac cycle. Therefore, collagen plays a major physiological role during contraction and relaxation by coupling the mechanical activity of the different contractile units (Table 2. 6). Each capillary is equally interconnected with surrounding myocytes by another type of struts (Figure 2. 16) whose role is to maintain the capillary flow during systole. The presence of a normal collagen matrix is essential during the development, and blocking collagen synthesis by treating newborn rats with β-aminopropionitril results in multiple areas of necrosis and aneurysm of the ventricle.

Table 2. 6. Physiological role of the myocardial and vascular collagen network [from Weber et al. 1993 and Tedgui et Levy 1994].

---

1. Connections between myocytes to maintain cardiovascular architecture,

2. Rigid network around the cardiac myocytes and the vascular wall to prevent excessive stretch,

3. Transmission of force generated by contractile elements to the chamber, and

4. Storage of energy during diastole in the heart and during diastole in the aorta (in the aorta, during diastole, energy is used to deliver blood to the periphery through the elastic fibers).

Collagen represents 3% of the myocardial mass. Myocardial collagen is routinely quantified by quantitative morphology or by measuring the amount of hydroxyproline, an amino acid specific for this protein. The myocardial collagen matrix consists primarily of type I collagen (85% of which aggregates into thick fibers) and type III collagen which forms thinner fibers and represents 11% of the total collagen content. Valve leaflets contain 20% type III collagen. Type IV collagen is a minor component and is included into arterial wall intima and also basal membrane of cardiomyocytes. Arterial walls contain type IV collagen in intima and cardiomyocytes posses. The media contains lamellar units, which are composed of muscle cells surrounded by elastic fibers made of elastin and maintained in order by collagen fibrils. As in the heart, the collagen is mainly types I and III.

Collagen I has the tensile strength of steel [Weber et al 1993]. Collagen plays a major physiological role as detailed in Table 2. 4. Collagen is a determinant of both ventricular and arterial stiffness, and the collagen content of the LV is correlated with the tissue compliance (which is calculated from the stress/strain relationships, as oposed to chamber compliance which is calculated from the pressure/volume curve). Cardiac fibrosis is due to an increased collagen concentration and occurs in 3 different conditions: senescence, after ischemia or under the influence of hormones (angio II, catecholamines, and aldosterone) [Weber et al. 1993]. It renders the myocardial tissue less compliant and more heterogeneous and favors arrhythmias. Fibronectins are another important component of the ECM both of the heart and the blood vessels. Fibronectin is a 500 kDa dimeric glycoprotein which originates either from exsudation of soluble plasma fibronectin (pFN), or from the local synthesis and secretion of a cellular form (cFN). Both forms are synthesized from a single gene and are composed of three types of repeats - types I, II and III. pFN and cFN differ in the number of their alternatively spliced sequences, the IIIA and B repeats being specific for cFN. The expression of these different forms of fibronectin are developmentally regulated and specifically reexpressed in adults in hypertrophied heart. FN has specific domains of binding to collagen and to cell receptors - namely integrins that are firmly attached to the cytoskeleton.

134

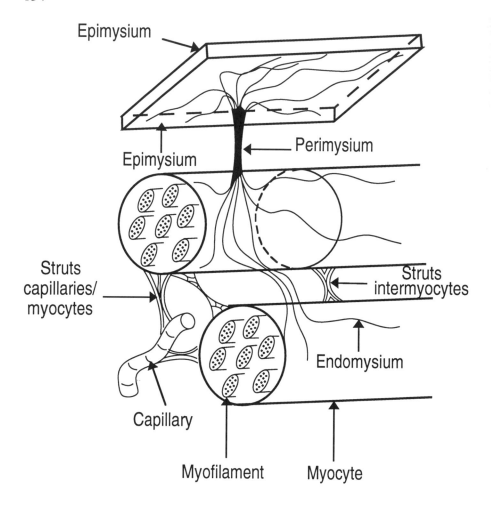

Fig. 2.16. Structure of the collagen network
[from Swynghedauw 1990, with permission].

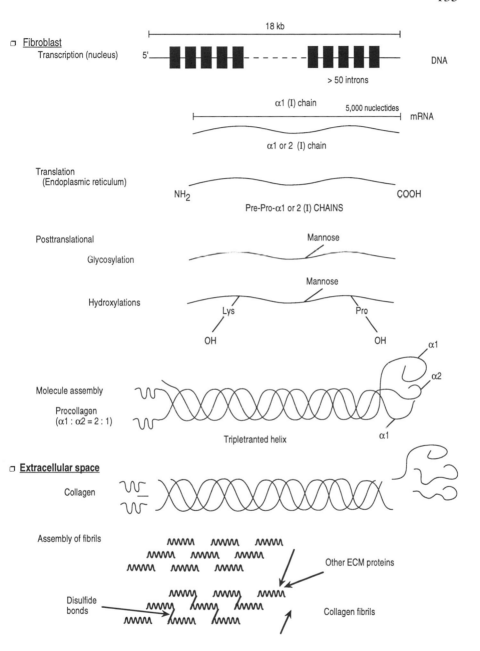

Fig. 2.17. Type I collagen synthesis

Collagen metabolism

Synthesis and degradation

Type I collagen is a long (300nm) and bulky heteropolymer, consisting of 3 chains (or subunits) - 2 $\alpha1(I)$ and one $\alpha2(I)$, which form a triple-helical domain. Each chain is made up of more than 1,000 amino acid residues. The genes encoding the $\alpha1$ and $\alpha2$ chains are different but similar in structure since they both contain more than 50 exons. In humans, the locus for $\alpha1$ is on chromosome 17 and consists of approximately 18 kb; the gene of $\alpha2$ is on chromosome 7 and consists of 38 kb of sequence.

Collagen is both synthesized and degraded by fibroblasts, and attempts to demonstrate collagen synthesis in myocytes have been unsuccessful. The biosynthesis of collagen is a rather complex phenomena and, at least in the cardiovascular system, consists of a poorly explored cascade of events (Figure 2. 17). Collagen half-life is unique with respect to its length, which is approximately 100 days, as compared to that of myosin, for example, which is around 7 days. In some tissues the half-life can even be much longer. This is due to both a slow rate of synthesis (0.56% per day in the ventricle) and degradation.

The initial translational products - prepro-$\alpha1$ (I) or 2 (I) chain - are translocated in the endoplasmic reticulum of the fibroblasts and cleaved into pro–$\alpha1$ (I) or 2 (I) chain. Then several posttranslational modifications take place, including hydroxylations and glycosylation. These modifications are a necessary prerequisite for stabilization of the structures and assembly of the chains into a molecule which is then secreted into the extracellular space to constitute fibrils in the extracellular matrix (Figure 2.21).

The packing of collagen molecules into fibrils is associated with the formation of covalent crosslinks between the molecules. The molecules are arranged in parallel and in register with respect to one another. They are

A

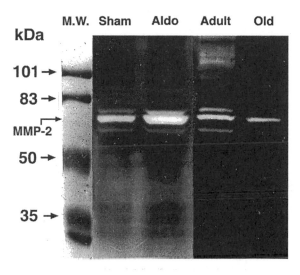

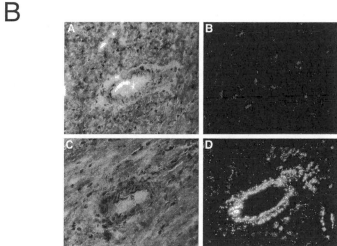

Fig. 2.18. Zymographic analysis of matrix metalloproteinases activities in rats. (A): SDS-PAGE gelatin zymographic electrophoresis. Left ventricular extracts. Left: sham-operated and 2-month aldosterone-salt treated rats. Right: adult as compared to senescent (old) animals. (B): Photomicrographs of coronary arteries. (A and C): eosin-hemaline coloration. (B and D): in situ zymography. Sham-operated: A and B. 2-Month aldosterone-salt treated animals: C and D [from Robert et al. 1997, with permission].

138

separated by regular gaps and assembled into a matrix that contains several other extracellular matrix molecules.

Collagenases

Collagenases - also called *Matrix metalloproteinases* (*MMP*) - are members of a multigene family which have been classified on the basis of their substrate specificity and secretion in zymogen form, a proecess requiring extracellular activation. MMP-1 cleaves collagen molecules at a single site in the native triple helix and generates three-fourth and one-fourth collagen fragments, also known as gelatins. Unfolded gelatin triple helix can be further degraded into smaller fragments or amino acids by MMP-2, which is also capable of degrading collagen-IV and fibronectin. Gelatin-polyacrylamide gel electrophoresis allows the simultaneous detection of major MMPs and measurement of their relative activity. The technique can be applied to histological detection of the enzymatic activity. In rat heart, MMP activities appear as a doublet (MW 72 and 68 kd) corresponding to latent and active proMMP-2, respectively. A fainter third band (MW 54 kd) corresponding to proMMP-1 is also observed (Figure 2. 18). MMP-1 is not constitutively expressed in the interstitium and the corresponding mRNA cannot be detected in the heart in normal conditions, in contrast to MMP-2 [Robert et al. 1997].

VASOACTIVE ENDOTHELIAL SUBSTANCES

Vascular tone is regulated by both the ANS and the vascular endothelium. There is, for the moment, a number of endothelial factors, which are mostly peptides, that play a role in the regulation of vascular function. Obviously some are still unknown and the list is far from being complete [Tedgui et Levy 1994]. More recently, it has been shown that most, if not all, of these

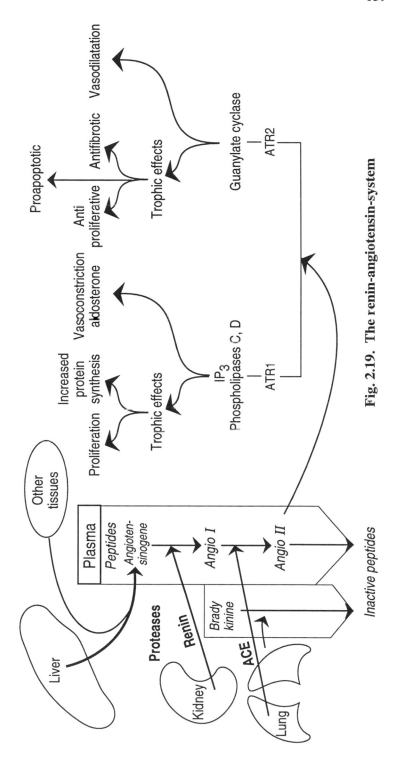

Fig. 2.19. The renin-angiotensin-system

vasoactive factors may also regulate myocardial function and possess a trophic effect.

The renin-angiotensin system (RAS)

This system is the most popular because of the discovery of 2 classes of drugs that interact with one of its components. Numerous symposia have also rendered the RAS very familar to clinicians. This area is a major target for pharmacological research and a major goal for detecting genetic abnormalities in essential hypertension. In addition, the recent discovery of various receptor subtypes and the trophic role of angiotensin II open new avenues for exploring the physiopathology of various cardiac diseases, including heart failure, myocardial infarction, and hypertensive macroangiopathy.

The RAS is a proteolytic pathway that transforms an inactive peptide, angiotensinogene (angne) into an active peptide, angio II. Angio II is a potent vasoconstrictor playing a major role in the physiological regulation of blood pressure (Figure 2.19). There is an intermediary step, which consists in the transformation of angne by a protease, renin, into a smaller peptide, angio I. Angio I is in turn degraded by a second metallopeptidase, angio I converting enzyme (ACE).

Structure of RAS Components

Angiotensinogene. The protein is a rather bulky globular protein (MW 55 to 65 kd) found in the plasma, and mainly synthesized in the pericentral zone of liver globules, but also in the atria and arterial wall (see below). The gene is unique and composed of 5 exons and encompasses 13 kb. The 5' flanking region of the gene contains three glucocorticoid responsive elements, a thyroid and an estrogen responsive element. These structural data were confirmed by physiological studies that demonstrated an increased plasma level of angne following stimulation by the above hormones. the liver content in angne mRNA increases after bilateral nephrectomy or when the plasma level of angio II is enhanced, nevertheless, as a rule for the different components of the RAS, angne mRNA is differentially regulated in various tissues.

Renin. Renin is a single chain 37 to40 kb glycoprotein enzyme found in plasma (routine quantification includes either immunological quantification of the protein or enzymatic detection of plasma renin activity) mainly synthesized in the juxtaglomerular apparatus in the afferent arterioles of the kidney. Renin is specific for angne and the unique enzyme responsible for transforming angne into angio I. The gene is unique in human (but in rats there are 2 genes), is composed of 10 exons, and encompasses 12.5 kb. During the first step of translation the renin mRNA first yields a preprorenin and then a prorenin that appears in the circulation where it is further transformed into renin. The 5' flanking region of the gene contains DNA consensus sequences specific for cAMP, glucocorticoid, estrogen, and progesterone, and the plasma level of renin is consequently hormonally regulated. The angne renin mRNA is differentially regulated in various tissues.

Angiotensin Converting Enzyme. ACE is a dipeptidyl metallo (that binds zinc to be activated) cardoxypeptidase.In contrast with renin, ACE is a rather nonspecific protease that not only transforms angio I into angio II, but also can degrade bradykinin into an inactive form. Consequently, ACE inhibition results not only in a lower plasma level of angio II, but also in an increased concentration in bradykinin which is a potent vasodilator. ACE exists as two different isoforms, the endothelial form (MW 140 to 160 kd) and the testicular form (MW 90 to 100 kd), which are encoded by two different isomRNAs (4.5-5 kb and 2.6 kb) that are transcribed by alternative splicing (and initiation) of a single gene. The gene is composed of at least 6 exons. The ACE gene has consensus DNA sequences specific for glucocorticoid and cAMP, and indeed physiological studies have demonstrated that the expression of the gene is hormonally regulated.

Angiotensin II Receptors. ATR are going to become a major target for therapy since several specific inhibitors have now been proposed. The availability of these compounds has provided definitive evidence for the heterogeneity of ATR: the ATR subtype 1 (ATR1) is specifically blocked by Losartan and subdivided into ATR1A and ATR B (both are coded by two different genes located on chromosomes 17 and 2 respectively), while ATR2 is inhibited by PD 123177, PD 123319, and CGP 42112A (the latter also has an agonist effect). Both belong to the R7G family. Rat and human hearts contain equivalent amounts of ATR1 and ATR2 (4 and 8 fmol/mg, respectively) [Heymes et al. 1998].

(1) ATR1 mediates vasoconstriction, aldosterone secretion, Angio II-induced water drinking and tachycardia and plays a crucial role in the physiological control of blood pressure. Blockade of ATR1 inhibits the trophic effects of angio II and prevents cardiac hypertrophy. Activation of ATR1 result in a biphasic increase of the calcium transient that corresponds to an initial release of calcium from the calcium stores and a further activation of the inward current. ATR1s are coupled to phospholipase C through a Gq protein and by so doing activate the phosphoinositol cycle and hydrolyze phosphatidylcholine which in turn mobilizes intracellular calcium concentration and reduces intracellular pH. They are also coupled to phospholipase A2 and D.

(2) ATR2 are present in adult tissues but are more abundant in embryonic and neonatal tissues. Studies with transgenic mice have shown that ATR2 can mediate a vasodilator effect. There are several studides on

isolated cells suggesting that ATR2 inhibits cell proliferation. Nevertheless, contradictory results performed *in vivo* have been obtained, which show that plasma angio II can activate vascular wall hypertrophy and fibrosis.

The kinin-kallicrein system

The system is very similar to the RAS and includes an active peptide called *bradykinin*, that has a potent endothelium-dependent vasodilatory effect. Circulating bradykinin is inactivated by ACE: therefore, converting enzyme inhibitors can inhibit bradykinin degradation and also produce vasodilatation through this additional mechanism. The precursor of bradykinin is kallicrein, which is synthesized in the kidney. This organ is the only one to produce and degrade kinins. The kinin-kallicrein system is likely to exist as a tissue system, as the RAS.

Endothelium-derived vasoactive factors

It is now wellestablished that a number of vasoactive factors indirectly induced vasodilatation or vasoconstriction through the release of substances produced by the vascular endothelium.

Endothelium-dependent relaxation plays a major physiological role in maintaining vascular tone. It is dominated by the effects of short-lived substance(s) produced as nitric oxide (NO released by several vasoactive factors by the endothelial cells and acting on smooth muscle guanylate cyclase. Acetylcholine, for example, indirectly induces vasodilatation but requires the presence of an intact endothelium. Prostacyclin formation (PGI_2) also plays a role in vasorelaxation, but this a minor role as compare to NO.

Endothelium-dependent contraction is much more complex and includes the production of a variety of different compounds, including endothelin and locally synthesized angio II but also prostaglandin H_2 and thromboxan A_2, which all are acting in a second step, but by different mechanisms, on smooth muscle cells. It may play a physiological role in maintaining the vascular tone. Nevertheless, for the moment, it seems mainly involved in pathological states.

Endothelium-dependent relaxation

Endothelial cells produce at least 3 relaxing factors, including NO (previously called endothelium-dependent relaxing factor), which is the most important, prostacyclin PGI_2 (Figure 2. 20), and a hyperpolarizing factor (EDHF). A clinician has to be aware of the recent developments of research in the field of NO because there are several drugs that act through such a mechanism - such as molsidomine for example which is a NO donor.

Nitric oxide (NO). NO is the major physiological regulator of systemic resistance vessels tone since inhibition of the NO production decreases local blood flow. Concordant observations suggest indeed that arterial blood pressure is continuously regulated by NO, which is formed and released from the arterial endothelium. In cardiovascular pharmacology NO is the compound directly responsible for coronary-dilatation induced by nitroprusside or indirectly responsible for vasorelaxation after treatment by nitroglycerine. NO has a potent vasodilatory effect, but is also a trophic factor that inhibits cell proliferation and is formed on demand by the action of NO synthase (NOS) [Dinerman et al. 1993; Shepherd and Katusic 1991; Kelly et al. 1996].

NOS catalyzes the conversion of L-arginine to L-citrulline in the presence of oxygen and NADPH. Three NOSs have been described so far, each the product of separate homologous genes. The gene structure displays several binding sites: for oxidative factors as NADPH and sites for heme and calmodulin. Constitutively expressed NOS isoforms include nNOS (or

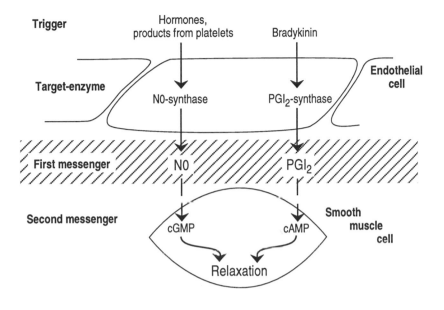

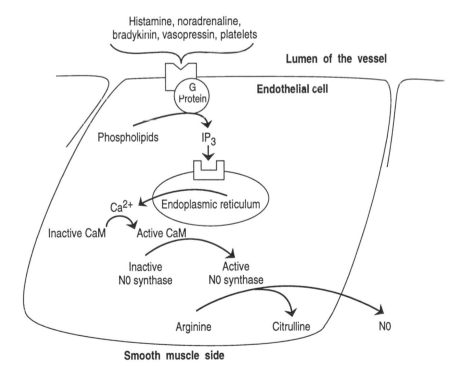

Fig. 2.20. Endothelial-dependent factors causing vasodilatation
Upper: endothelial cascade, lower: NO production

146

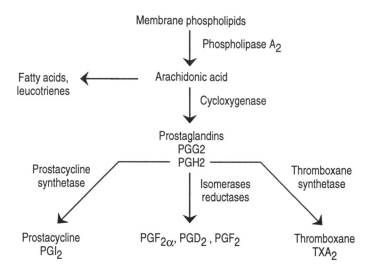

Fig. 2.21. **Metabolism of arachidonic acid and prostaglandins**

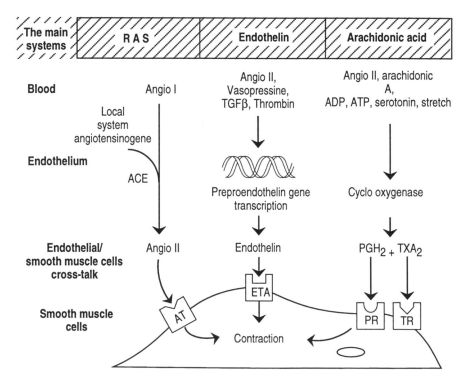

Fig. 2.22. **Endothelial-dependent factors causing vasoconstriction**

NOS1), the neuronal cytosolic form, and eNOS (or NOS3), the vascular endothelial form of which is associated to membranes. These isoforms are regulated by physiological concentrations of calcium. In contrast, cytokine-(and lipopolysaccharide-, cytokines include TNFα, interleukines, interferon) inducible iNOS (or NOS2) is insensitive to calcium and located into cytosol or particulate fractions. The heart does contain the 3 NOS isoforms [Kelly et al. 1996]. NO itself may regulate NOS expression and activity through the formation of ferrous-nitrosyl complexes in their heme prosthetic groups that self-inactivate these enzymes. NO is generated in the endothelial cells and released into the extracellular space.

In endothelial cells, NOS is activated by shear-stress and by various compounds, including acetylcholine, bradykinine, histamine, arginine, vasopressine, norepinephrine and several substances released by platelets, which all enhance intracellular calcium concentration through a cascade of events which involves the phosphoinositol cycle and the IP3 production (Figures 2. 21 and 2. 22). IP3 binds to an IP3 receptor on the endoplasmic reticulum and then releases calcium from endogenous stores as explained above (this important mechanism is reviewed in detail by Williamson and Monck [1992]). NOS is a phosphorylatable enzyme and can be phosphorylated by a cAMP-dependent protein kinase C that attenuates the enzyme activity. The most important target of NO is the soluble guanylate cyclase in smooth muscle cells. NO stimulates this cyclase as a consequence of the reaction of NO with the haem prosthetic group of the cyclase to form nitrosohaem. The result is an over 50-fold greater rate of cGMP synthesis than that catalysed by unnitrosylated cyclase. cGMP elicits muscle relaxation through its influence on calcium release from the endoplasmic reticulum and calcium influx through receptor-operated calcium channels. In addition to its vasorelaxing effect, NO exerts several important functions. It inhibits platelet aggregation and adhesion, modulates smooth muscle proliferation, generation of endothelin, and leucocytes and monocytes adhesion to endothelium, and finally is a potent antiatherosclerotic agent [Zeiher 1996].

Other vasodilating substances. Prostacyclin PGI_2 is another less important short-lived relaxing factor released by the endothelium. It is the major product of the metabolism of arachidonic acid by cyclooxygenase, and its endothelial production is also activated by various factors including thrombin, bradykinin, or shear stress (Figure 2. 22). The physiological effects of prostacyclin are mediated by cAMP. Nevertheless, inhibition of prostacyclin production, unlike inhibition of NO production, does not have any substantial effect on blood flow.

Differences exist between arteries and veins and even from one region to another. For example, thrombin relaxes large epicardial arteries in dogs by releasing EDRF, while it constricts the deep coronary resistance vessels and contracts veins.

Endothelium-dependent contraction

Endothelial cells produce and release several vasoconstricting substances that act through, at least, several different pathways: the RAS, cyclooxygenase-dependent endothelium-derived contracting factors, endothelin (Figure 2. 22) and pO_2 [Katusic and Sheperd 1991; Lüscher et al. 1992].

Endothelin. Preproendothelin is encoded by a gene located on chromosome 6 in humans and is sequentially transformed to proendothelin and then to endothelin by an endothelin converting enzyme [Lotersztajn 1993]. This is again a major target for pharmacological research in cardiology. Endothelin is a 21-residue peptide and its production is transcriptionally regulated and activated by thrombine, cytokines, epinephrine, vasopressine, angio II, endotoxine, and shear stress forces [Yanagisawa et al. 1988]. ANF and relaxing factors such as NO and prostacyclin reduce its production. There are

3 different isoendothelins - called 1, 2 and 3 - that are encoded by 3 different isogenes. Endothelin is different from angio II in terms of its vasoconstrictor effects since a single injection of endothelin results in a rapid and short episode of vasodilatation followed by a long-lasting period of hypertension for 2 to 3 hours. The receptors are G protein-dependent receptors containing 7 spanning domains and belong to the R7G family described above. The ET_A receptor is located on smooth muscles cell and is responsible for endothelin-induced vasoconstriction. By contrast, the ET_B receptor is on endothelial cells, activates NO synthase or IGI_2 formation, and is responsible for the short episode of vasodilation. The second messenger pathway is rather complex since endothelin and the corresponding endothelin receptors may act through nearly all the known pathways including cAMP production, PI cycle, and arachidonic acid (Figure 2. 25). Inhibitors of endothelin are now available for pharmacological applications. It is very unlikely that endothelin plays a role in maintaining blood pressure since inhibition of proendothelin production has no effect on blood pressure, but it certainly does play a role in pathological conditions.

Other vasoconstricting substances. Inhibitors of cyclooxygenase, such as indomethacin, can block endothelium-dependent contractions. Conversely, endothelial-dependent contractions can be induced by arachidonic acid, stretch, serotonin, or even by acetylcholine (which is normally a vasodilator) in arteries from spontaneously hypertensive rats (SHR).

Endothelial cells/cardiocytes cross-talk

This new area of research recently has received considerable attention. Pioneer works (reviewed in Brutsaert and Andries 1992) have clearly demonstrated that the selective destruction of the endocardium induced abbreviation of isometric twitch duration, with isometric force declining

150

sooner during relaxation. Both a release of endocardial substances with inotropic properties and a transendocardial endothelial physicochemical control are postulated as possible underlying mechanisms. Endocardial and coronary endothelia are also likely to play an important role in the regulation of cardiac hypertrophy.

THE HEART AND VESSELS AS ENDOCRINES

Atrial natriuretic peptides (ANP)

The first demonstration of the regulation of the atrial system by modifications in sodium balance or volume was done by Pierre Yves Hatt in Limeil-Brevannes, France, who demonstrated that sodium restriction results in an increased granular appearance in the atria, whereas high sodium diet, desoxycorticosterone, or chronic volume overload decreases granulation density [Marie et al. 1976]. The atrial natriuretic factor (ANF) was further identified and the corresponding gene cloned. ANF gene is located on chromosome 1 in humans, and translated into a preproANF and a proANF. In humans active ANF is in a 28 aminoacid peptide that is stored in granulations as a propeptide. In adult mammals, the ANF mRNA is quite abundant in both right and left atria and rare in other tissues. ANF production is developmentally regulated, and the ventricular level of ANF mRNA during embryogenesis is comparable to that of atria in adults. ANF production is activated by atrial distension but also by several hormones such as glucocorticoids and thyroid hormone. Mechanical volume overload in atria and pressure overload in ventricles induce the production of ANF mRNA and secretion of the peptide by the myocardium. The putative regulatory region was located 2.5 kb upstream of the coding part of the gene.

ANF is a potent diuretic that enhances natriuresis by decreasing the proximal tubule reabsorption of sodium and inhibiting aldosterone production. In addition, ANF has a vasodilator activity. Thus it opposes nearly every effect of angio II. ANF exerts its effects through specific receptors and the cGMP pathway.

Myocardial and vascular RAS

Converting enzyme inhibition is still capable of lowering blood pressure after blocking circulating angio II with appropriate antibodies which suggests that tissue RAS is present and functional. Tissue RAS has been directly evidenced in both vessels and myocardium: in the heart, positive immunoreactivity for angiotensinogen has been found predominantly in atria and double immunogold labeling has shown that ANF is located in specific granules and angiotensinogen is present on both granules and myofibrils. The ACE, which is a membrane-bound protein, and renin have also been successfully evidenced in the myocardium, although renin is rare, or even absent, in the ventricles. As a final result, isolated hearts produce angiotensinogen and angiotensin II.

The human heart differs from that of rat in terms of tissue RAS, and its production of angiotensin II uses two different pathways - namely, the ACE, which predominates in atria, and an angiotensin II-forming chymase which predominates in the ventricles [Urata et al. 1993]. The functional significance of the abovefindings have been confirmed by showing a partial inhibition in the formation of angiotensin II in the human heart by CEI.

Direct assessment of angiotensin I and II levels in canine myocardial interstitial fluid were obtained by using microdialysis probes and showed levels >100-fold higher than plasma levels that are not affected by intravenous angiotensin II nor CEI suggesting that angiotensin II production or degradation in the heart is compartmentalized and mediated by different mechanisms than in intravascular spaces [Dell'Italia et al. 1997]. The functional role of the tissular RAS is likely to be of minor importance in normal conditions. Nevertheless, this system may play a more significant role under pharmacological influences or during aging [Heymes et al. 1994).

Aldosterone, corticosterone and a few other compounds

The heart also possess an endocrine steroidogenic system. There is now evidence that the heart contains the main enzymes responsible for aldosterone synthesis - namely, 11β-hydroxylase and aldosterone synthase - and that isolated hearts produce aldosterone, corticosterone, and deoxycorticosterone. This production is regulated by sodium diet, angio II and ACTH. Myocardial aldosterone production could counteract the effects of ANF [Silvestre et al. 1998]. Recently it has also been shown that the heart is able to produce vasopressine and possess adrenergic cells, which constitutively release catecholamines.

CARDIAC AND VASCULAR GROWTH

Every step of the cardiac development is characterized by a specific genetic program. A major switch from the foetal to adult program occurs the first week after birth, and there is compelling evidences that cardiac and vascular hypertrophy phenotypes in adults reproduce such a foetal program, as initially demonstrated in our laboratory [Lompré et al. 1979]. Cardiac hypertrophy is a clinical problem of crucial importance that is described in detail in the next chapter. Vascular hypertrophy is equally important. It is now well-documented that the vascular wall thickens in response to chronic arterial hypertension, which constitutes both an important risk factor and a major target for drug therapy.

Cardiac, arterial, and arteriolar hypertrophy of pathological origin results from the abnormal triggering of the normal growth process. It is therefore important to know the main avenues used by the cardiovascular system for growth and development. The topic is becoming popular and the amount of informations relative to growth signals in the heart and in the arteries is increasing every month. A major problem in this field of investigation comes from the complexity of the situation. Both pure mechanics and hormones or peptides may influence cell growth and proliferation and protein synthesis, and it is sometimes impossible to know what is really determinant in the growth process. The question is far from being academic since the 2 factors are accessible to therapeutic intervention.

It is usual to describe the process of growth in 3 steps: the triggers, the growth pathways, and the targets (Figure 2. 23) [Swynghedauw 1986, van Bilsen and Chien 1991; Tedgui et Levy 1994]. These steps are remarkably similar both in the heart and the vessels and involve transcription. Nevertheless, there are also processes that are posttranscriptionally regulated: for the moment these have been only poorly documented.

Cellular growth

Cardiac myocytes are terminally differentiated cells incapable of division in adults. In humans, cardiac hypertrophy induced by mechanical overload is due to an increase in the size of the cardiocytes with an unchanged number of the cells, in the same condition. Nonmuscular cells (endothelial, fibroblasts, and macrophages) increase both in number and size. Adult cardiocytes never, or rarely, divide (in fact, ancient and very recent investigations have suggested that mitosis can occur in adult cardiocytes during ischemia [Quaini et al. 1994]), at least by mitosis, whereas nonmuscle cells are still able to produce mitotic figures. Growth during the foetal period or childhood is different and results from both hyperplasia and hypertrophy of all cells, including the cardiocytes.

Vascular endothelial cells are able to replicate in the adult. Smooth muscle cells of the small arteries usually become hyperplasic when submitted to mechanical stress. By contrast, the same cells in the aorta areunable to divide, and the response to mechanical overload is hypertrophy without cell division. Nevertheless, such a phenotypic response depends on the experimental conditions, and there are conditions during which smooth muscle cells of the aorta can also proliferate [Tedgui et Levy 1994].

Triggers and pathways for growth

By *trigger*, we mean every event able to initiate the process such as stretch or mechanical activity (termed *mechanotransduction*), hormones, or peptides. Triggers produce a signal that is transduced from the membrane to the nucleus and then activates transcription and produces hypertrophy. Growth factors are not stricto sensu triggers (except in certain experimental conditions) since their expression is mostly triggered by various compounds.

Mechanical factors
In many biological systems mechanical forces regulate genetic expression: in bacteria changes in turgor pressure induce osmoregulatory genes: in plants both gravity and wind regulate growth; in mammalians stretching an axon, a fibroblast, or a myocyte activates growth. The mechanogenetic regulation of transcription is far from being simple and is likely to involve different pathways, including mechanosensory channels, stretch receptors, the direct effect of stretch on membrane phospholipases, and the cytoskeleton itself [reviewed in Erdös et al. 1991].

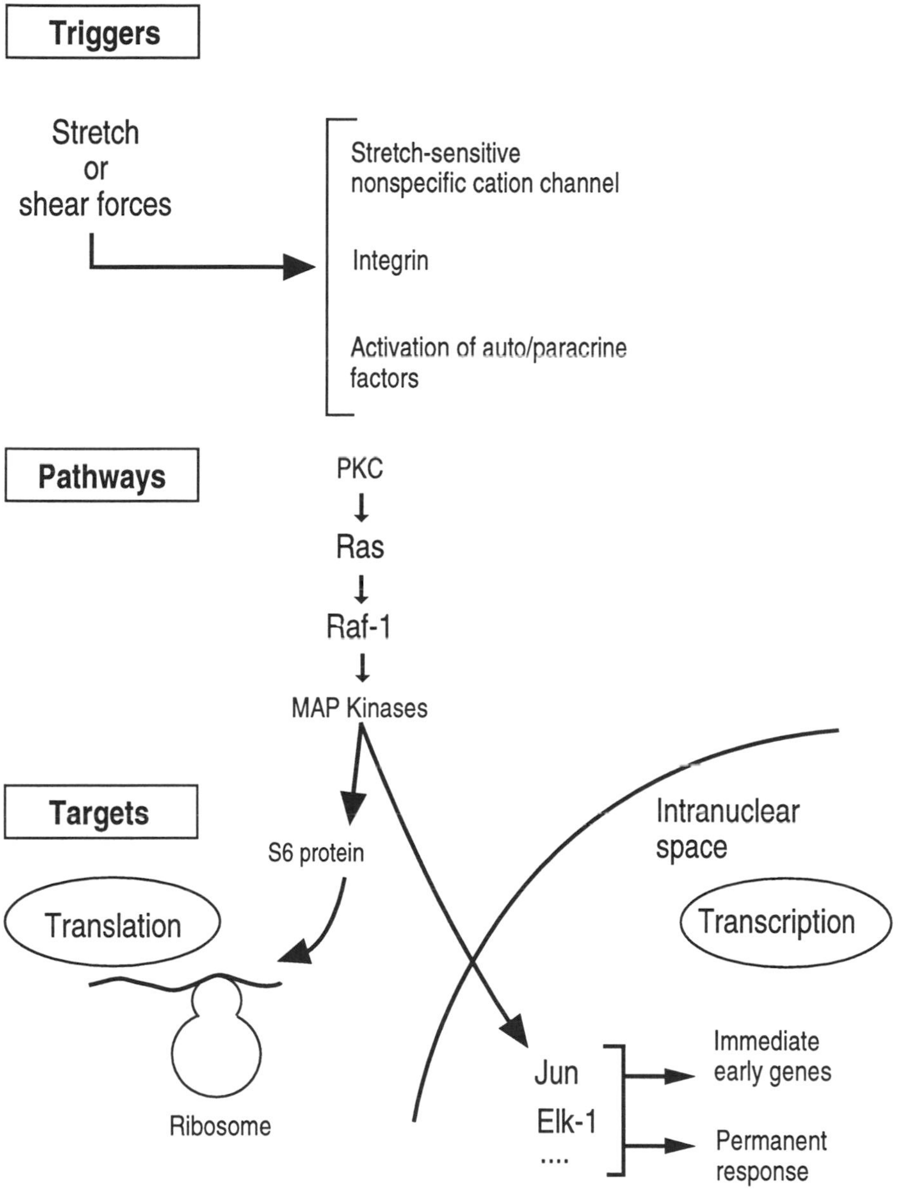

Fig. 2.23. The biological cascades at the origin of
cardiac or vascular hypertrophy

Mechanical forces obviously are specific triggers for muscle growth and indeed play a role in myometrium, vessels and myocardium. For example, in skeletal muscle passive stretch, such as that obtained by bilateral removal of the insertion of the tendon of the distal portion of the synergistic gastrocnemius muscle, results in an activation of protein synthesis and a differential modification of the expression of the gene coding for myosin isoforms in the controlateral muscles. Passive stretch of the heart both activates protein synthesis and modulates myocardial gene expression in isolated adult and neonatal cardiocytes, in papillary muscle, and also on coronary perfused heart (in the latter, stretch is obtained through the Gregg's effect - that is sarcomere stretching due to an excessive coronary distension) [Delcayre et al. 1992].

The endothelium plays a particular role in this process. Endothelium is located at the interface between blood flow and the vascular or cardiac wall and functions as a mechanical sensor that is permanently exposed to pressure and stretch forces as well as high fluid shear stress [Davies and Tripathi 1993]. Nevertheless, endothelium is not unique in responding to mechanical forces, and nearly every cell accommodates to such a trigger. Blood flow regulates the internal diameter of vessels both acutely by vasomotricity and chronically by the reorganization of vascular wall cellular and extracellular components.

Mechano-sensing is still a controversial issue: (1) pressure stretch can activate several ion channels, including a nonspecific cation channel that can be blocked by gadolinium and streptomycine and a gadolinium-insensitive stretch-activated K^+ channel: such channels are likely to play a role in the genesis in the arrhythmias which are triggered by acute cardiac distension; (2) shear stretch on endithelial cells activates the formation of endothelin-1, bFGF, and NO and then can modify nuclear transcription; (3) recent evidence suggests that the cytoskeleton through integrins and focal adhesion kinases may act as a sensor, which could elicit tyrosine kinase phosphorylation and therefore mechanically transduce the mechanical signal to the genome; (4) another possibility would involve the mechanically induced production of a variety of hormones, including the myocardial or vascular RAS, and endothelin or cytokines (growth factors) through autocrine or paracrine mechanisms.

Hormones and peptides

Several hormones, nearly every vasoactive peptides and most of the growth factors possess a trophic effect in addition to their known physiological function:

Stimulation of α1-adrenergic receptors by norepinephrine is coupled to the transcription of genes encoding early developmental isoforms of contractile proteins (β-myosin heavy chain and skeletal α-actin) and *c-myc* in the cardiocytes. The intracellular pathway connecting the a1-receptor to the genome probably involves the phospholipase C (PFC) -dependent phosphorylation of a specific transcription factor [Simpson et al. 1990].

β1-adrenergic stimulation has also, in certain experimental conditions, a specific trophic effect and stimulates noncontractile protein synthesis in isolated adult cardiocytes [Dubus et al. 1990].

The trophic effect of thyroid hormones is well documented and includes both hypertrophy and a differential activation of several isogenes. Thyroxine activates the expression of several genes, including a-myosin heavy chain and β-adrenergic receptor.

Angio II induces the growth response and stimulates cell proliferation in smooth muscle cells grown in serum, suggesting that such a proliferative effectrequires the presence of other factors, and indeed angio II amplifies the proliferative response to EGF or PDGFB. It has mainly a direct hypertrophic effect through the well-known enhancer element, AP1. The activation of this enhancer depends on protein kinase C pathway. angio II induces the expression of *c-myc*, *c-fos*, PDGF A and TGF β. The determinants of the trophic effects of Angiotensin II are quite complex, since angio II can activate both a proliferative and an antiproliferative pathway through ATR1 and ATR2 (see above angio II receptors, (ATRs). Converting enzyme inhibition is known to prevent both vascular fibrosis and hypertrophy and to have an effect on cardiac hypertrophy, which is, in part, independent from the effect on blood pressure.

Intracellular signaling pathways

Many different pathways are activated in response to different hypertrophic stimuli. Several cross-links are well characterized between these pathways, and the scheme is becoming an incredibly complicated puzzle [Swynghedauw and Coraboeuf 1994; Shiojima et al. 1996; Hefti et al. 1997].

The mitogen-activated protein kinase (MAP kinase), pathway is the best documented pathway that can mediate both the stretch-induced hypertrophy and the trophic effects of angiotensin II. (1) Transfection experiments have demonstrated that the PKC is involved in the strech-induced expression of several oncogenes through a consensus DNA sequence located upstream the oncogene and called serum responsive element. PKC isoforms might be the second messenger in the signaling pathway between both the mechanical stimulus and angiotensin II, and the nuclear response. (2) PKC is a kinase, which in turn phosphorylates a low molecular weight GTP-binding protein, *p21 Ras* and then a cascade of phosphorylations of another group of kinases, including *Raf-1* (which is an oncogene), MAPKKK, MAPKK, and MAPK. (3) The last component of this cascade translocates into the nucleus where it activates transcription through *Jun*, *Elk-1* and other *oncogenes*.

The receptors of most growth factors are transmembrane tyrosine kinases (Figure 2. 24). When activated by the ligand, the receptors phosphorylate themselves (autophosphorylation) at specific intracellular sites and bind specifically several signalling proteins, including phosphatidylinositol 3-kinase, which activate mitogenesis: the γ isoform of phospholipase C, which activates phosphatidylinositol hydrolysis and consequently increases the $[Ca]_i$; and GTP-bound *Ras*. *Ras* plays a central role and transmits the signal through several pathways including the MAP kinase pathway, the mitogen-activated extracellular signal regulated kinase (MEK) pathway and several others [von Harsdorf et al. 1989; Hefti et al. 1997].

The cytoskeleton proteins, as shown above, are also likely to be a pathway, and integrin-linked microfilaments together with other components of the cytoskeleton can transduce the stress to the nucleus directly or through the secretion of growth factors.

Transcription factors (TF)

Genetic control of cardiac development

It is possible to "oblige" an undifferentiated cell, or nearly so, such as a fibroblast, to become a differentiated cell, like a myoblast, by introducing a single factor. Such factors are nuclear proteins termed *transcription factors* (TFs). TFs bind specific consensus DNA sequences usually located within the gene promotor and act on the transcriptional process to coordinate the expression of several genes in order to make an entirely new differentiated cell. The best example is MyoD. MyoD, when injected into a fibroblast, is able to transform this cell into a fully differentiated skeletal myocyte: nevertheless, MyoD is absent from the heart.

In contrast to skeletal muscle, the genetic program regulating cardiac development is complex, combinatorial, and multifactorial [Harvey et al. 1997; Grépin et al. 1995]. There are, for the moment, three TFs that have been identified in the heart: (1) CATF, which binds the specific DNA consensus sequence CARE and transactivates ANF gene expression; (2)

MEF2, which belongs to the MADS motif family, interacts with other TF (Nk2.5, and MHox), and regulates the expression of the gene encoding a specific cardiac myosin light chain. (3) The GATA motif is present on a variety of zinc-finger TF, and there is now evidence that GATA4 plays an important role during the process of cardiac hypertrophy. A GATA4 motif is present on both the promoter of the myosin heavy chain β and that of the angiotensin receptor subtype 1A. Direct injection of this promoter + various mutagenesis experiments were made after aortic banding in rats and demonstrate that GATA4 mediates the hypertrophic responsiveness. It also regulates the expression of ANF, brain natriuretic peptides, myosin and the cardiac TNC isoform during development. For the moment, GATA4 is the only TF so far described that directly regulates cardiac hypertrophy.

Other potential candidates include (1) a DNA binding dimerization motif termed helix-loop-helix (HLH) which is linked to a basic region, bHLH, this motif is found in MyoD1, myogenin, E12 and E47; (2) the leucine zipper (bZIP) that binds DNA to protooncogenes such as *c-myc, c-jun* and *c-fos*, but also to the cAMP-responsive element binding protein (CERB). (3) The helix-turn-helix (HTH) motif is found in homeoprotein and SOX; and (4) activator protein 2 (AP2) and the serum responsive factor are also transcriptional factors that play an important role in the cardiovascular system.

Nuclear hormone receptors

Several transcriptional factors specific for hormonal transduction, including CRE (Fig. 1. 11) have also been described, and several amino acid sequences able to bind specific DNA sequences have been reported.

Activated protein kinases modulate the function of TF, which binds a consensus sequence TGACGTCA, the CRE, in the regulatory region of genes sensitive to cAMP, and indirectly to adrenergic hormones. The coresponding protein, CREB, belongs to the basic region/leucine zipper TF class that is characterized by a DNA-binding domain composed of 30 basic amino acids. A heptad leucine repeat close to this domain can form amphiphatic α-helices with leucine residues aligned along one ridge associating in a coiled-coil conformation (leucine zipper), forming finally a dimer. The dimer juxtaposes the basic region and forms a particular Y-shaped structure that has the property to wrap around the major groove of the DNA Watson's helix [Watson et al. 1987]. Interestingly, the expression of the gene encoding the above-described TF is autoregulated by a sort of feedback mechanism by the Inducible cAMP Early Repressor that is involved in circadian rhythms [reviewed in Lalli and Sassone-Corsi 1994]. The hypertrophic response that is induced by adrenergic ligands is likely to be mediated by CREB.

Thyroxine, glucocorticoid, mineralocorticoid, progesterone and estrogen receptors are all part of a large family of intracellular hormone receptors that share a common general structure, including a central highly conserved DNA binding site of about 70 amino acids, a C-terminal steroid recognition region, and a finger-like structure that is activated in the presence of an atom of zinc (Table 2. 1) [Evans 1988]. These receptors are in fact true TFs, which bind to the corresponding consensus DNA sequence located upstream from gene. The thyroxine receptor is also an oncogene, called *c-erb-A*, and has a particular interest in cardiology since there are positive and negative thyroxine responsive elements in the regulatory region of genes coding for adrenergic receptors, cardiac isoforms of myosin heavy chains, phospholamban and so on.

The mineralo (or type I aldosterone receptor) and glucocorticoid (type II) receptors demonstrate a poor selectivity between glucocorticoids and aldosterone. Aldosterone only interacts with the mineraloreceptor type I because, in the aldosterone target tissue, this class of receptor is associated with 11-β-hydroxy-steroid dehydrogenase (11βHSD), an enzymatic complex that transforms cortisol into an inactive form unable to bind to the receptor.

Both types of receptors, and also the 11βHSD, are present in the myocytes of the myocardium. Aldosterone activates several plasma membrane channels, exchangers, or enzymes in the kidney and also has an effect on the transcription of these components. Aldosterone could have a determinant role during fibrogenesis [Brilla et al. 1990; Robert et al. 1994, 1997].

Early transitory DNA responses

Both mechanical stress and hormonal signals elicit an early transitory increase in the expression of several groups of genes, called immediate early genes, including protooncogenes, stress proteins and cytokines.

Protooncogenes

Initially the term *oncogene (onc)* was used to qualify genes able to induce cancer in experimental conditions in eucaryotes (Table 2. 7). The first oncogenes to be discovered were viral and termed *v-onc*. Later, it was demonstrated that onc exists in normal conditions and encodes numerous proteins playing a role in cell growth: they are termed *proto* or *cellular oncogenes*. The definition of oncoproteins is vague and in fact includes proteins that have diverse functions but may become transforming when modified. Nuclear *c-onc* mRNAs, including the *c-fos/c-jun* or *c-fos/AP1* nucleoprotein complex and *c-myc*, are transiently expressed when protein kinase C is activated or intracellular calcium or cAMP concentrations are enhanced both during embryonic development and also after an acute mechanical overload or hormonal stimulation, in the heart and vessels [Bauters et al. 1988; Izumo et al. 1988]. Whether or not these transcripts are also translated into oncoproteins, at least during mechanical overload, is still controversial [Snoeckx et al. 1991]. These oncoproteins bind DNA and confer competence to the cell to express a new genetic program.

Table 2. 7. Major protooncogenes. (Chr. 5, 7, 17 indicates chromosomal localization in humans).

Cytosolic *c-onc*

With tyrosine Kinase activity

c-erb-B: EGF receptor (Chr. 7)

c-*fms*: CSF1 receptor (Chr 5q34)

c-src: inhibits differentiation (Chr 20q12)

Transducers (GTPases)

c-Ki-ras2, c-Ha-ras1 (Chr 11): activate PLC

Others

c-erb-A: thyroid hormone receptor (Chr 17)

c-sis: PDGF B (Chr 22)

Nuclear *c-onc*

c-fos (Chr 14) and c-jun

c-myc (Chr 8q24)

Cytokines

Cytokines are a family of glycoproteins nonimmunoglogulin in nature acting nonenzymatically in pico or nanomolar concentration by interacting with specific receptors, which mostly belong to the tyrosine kinase family (Figure 2. 24). Cytokines mostly exert an effect on cell proliferation and biosynthesis and for this reason are frequently considered as synonymous of growth factors (GF) [Cummins 1993]. Nevertheless, cytokines have functions other than growth. In addition, distinct cytokines often exhibit similar biological activities.

GF are a polymorphic group of polypeptides that includes genuine GF, such as EGF or TGF, but also some hormones - for example insulin,

164

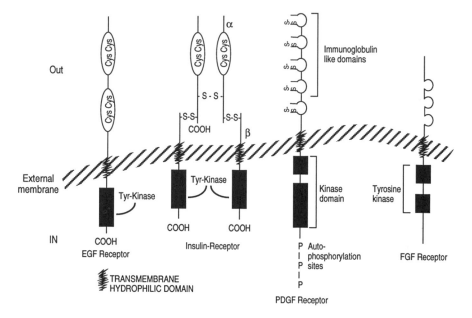

Fig. 2.24. Tyrosine kinase receptors

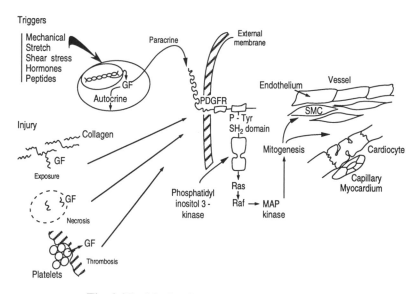

Fig. 2.25. Mechanisms of action of growth factors (GF)

Table 2. 8. Main families of growth factors.

Epithelial growth factor (EGF)

Mitogenic, stimulates angiogenesis, endothelial cell proliferation, and migration;

EGF, transforming growth factor-α (TGF-α) (MW 6,000 Da)*;

Receptor with cytoplasmic tyrosine kinase activity;

Distribution: wide.

Platelet-derived growth factor (PDGF)

Mitogenic, facilitates capillary formation;

Heterodimer (AA, AB, BB, MW 14 and 17,000 Da), vascular endothelial growth factor (VEGF);

Receptor with tyrosine kinase activity;

Distribution: wide, endothelial, PDGF is also a chemoattractant for neutrophils.

Fibroblast (or heparin-binding) growth factor (FGF)

Mitogen for fibroblasts and vascular endothelium, promotes angiogenesis (proliferation, migration, and organization of endothelial cells);

Acidic and basic FGF, aFGF and bFGF (MW 15 to 17,000 Da);

Distribution: very wide for bFGF, limited for a FGF, bFGF binds heparan sulphate glycosaminoglycans in ECM and is stored there, FGF 3 to 7.

Transforming growth factor-β (TGF-β)

Can promotes, but usually inhibits growth, development and angiogenesis, stimulates ECM formation;

TGF-β 1, 2, 3 (homodimer, MW 25,000 Da)*;

Receptors: transmembrane proteins with Serine/Threonine Kinase;

Distribution: universal.

Others

Insulin-like growth factor (IGF): receptor with tyrosine kinase activity;

Insulin: IGF-I, IGF-II;

Interleukins (IL): IL receptors; IL 1 to 8;

Colony stimulatory factor (CSF): interleukin receptors or receptors with tyrosine kinase;

Tumor necrosis factor (TNF): TNF α and β;

Neuropeptides: R7G; vasopressin, endothelin, gastrin-releasing peptide.

---

*TGF-β and TGF-α are unrelated molecules.

which has a trophic effect in addition to its known effect on glycemia - and vasoactive peptides such as endothelin and angiotensin II (Table 2. 8).

These polypeptides can be either induced by mechanical stretch, shear stress, hormones, or peptides (there are also GFs that induce the synthesis of other GFs); released from blood cells as platelets or neutrophils; exposed during injury (FGF for example is linked to the ECM); released by necrotic cells (Figure 2. 25). GF are then allowed to bind specific receptors that are tyrosine kinases (Figure 2. 24).

Stress or heat-shock proteins (HSP)

HSP were initially described as proteins expressed during heat shock and whose expression protects the cellular components against further agression. HSP may bind mRNAs and prevent RNA lysis. The group includes several members of various MW. HSP 70 (MW 70,000) is induced by heating and ischemia in both the aorta and the myocardium, and by mechanical overload in the heart [Delcayre et al. 1988]. The group also includes ubiquitin (MW 7,600) which is cofactor for proteases and plays a role in the normal process of proteolysis.

HSP is likely to become a major marker for ischemia. There is an actual consensus that favors the role of these proteins as a myocardial protective agent that is responsible for myocardial preconditionning.

Permanent responses of the genome

The biological cascade describes above can occur during pathological events, such as arterial hypertension, or in more physiological conditions, including embryonic development, normal growth, aging, or training. It has now become more and more evident that in every case the cell utilizes the same genetic programme as the fetal one. The fetal program includes the general process of activation of every gene implicated in cell hypertrophy, induction of some gens that are expressed only in the fetus, like ANF in the ventricle, more specific changes as shifts in isogene expression (such as isomyosins, isoforms of Na^+, K^+-ATPase, lactate deshydrogenase and creatine kinase), or even the noninduction of the expression of certain genes resulting in a dilution of the corresponding protein and mRNA in the hypertrophied tissue (Ca^{2+}ATPase of SR, ryanodine receptor, β1-adrenergic and muscarinic receptors in certain conditions) [Swynghedauw and Corabocuf 1994; Shiojima et al. 1996]. Such a general process is not applicable to every biological component of the cardiovascular system and is different, at least for fibrogenesis and also angiogenesis.

Fibrogenesis is a major problem in cardiology both in the heart and vessels. It results from an accumulation of collagen that can be due to an enhanced synthesis or a decreased degradation; both of these phenomena occur in fibroblasts. Connective tissue infiltration by inflammatory cells play a central role at the beginning of the fibrotic process - for example, after ischemia. The activity of these cells in inducing fibrosis is mediated by several growth factors that activate either fibroblast proliferation or collagen synthesis and/or degradation [Maquart et al. 1994]: (1) EGF, PDGF, insulin growth factor-1, interleukin-1, FGF, and endothelin-1 can all activate fibroblast proliferation and are secreted by inflammatory cells; (2) collagen synthesis can be activated by IGF-1, several interleukins, and endothelin, but the best-known activator is TGF-β, a 25 kD homodimeric polymorphic protein that can be synthesized by nearly all the cells; TGF-β both activates the transcription of collagen and fibronectin genes and inhibits matrix degradation; (3) conversely there are several cytokines, such as tumor necrosis factor–α and relaxin, that inhibit collagen or fibronectin synthesis.

With angiogenesis a commonly accepted scheme is the following [Schott and Morrow 1993]: (1) GF are induced or exposed by injury (after a myocardial infarction), or released from various cells, (2) then bFGF, PDGF, and EGF bind to specific receptors, and the corresponding signal is then transduced via tyrosine kinase activity, and (3) and endothelial cells finally are allowed to divide and proliferate and sprouts of neovessels appear.

CELL DEATH

Cell death is an important determinant of cell development. The organism has to suppress fetal cells to develop the adult program. Cell death is also a continuous process that is finally responsible for senescence. During ischemia, cardiac remodelling, and cardiac failure, the amount of cell loss is directly related to cardiac function, reparative fibrosis, and compensated cardiac hypertrophy. Cell death can occur by two different, nearly opposed, processes - namely necrosis or apoptosis (Figure 2. 26).

Necrosis results from acute cellular ischemic injury and usually occurs in an area of contiguous cell that are perfused by the same coronary artery. It induces cell and cell organelles swelling and lysis. The intracellular contents released by necrosis provoke an inflammatory response. Necrosis is characterized by severe membrane alterations and is preceded by a period of time during which the diseased cells become permeable to immunoglobulins such as radioactive monoclonal antibodies rised against myosin. Uninjured cells   remain   unlabeled.

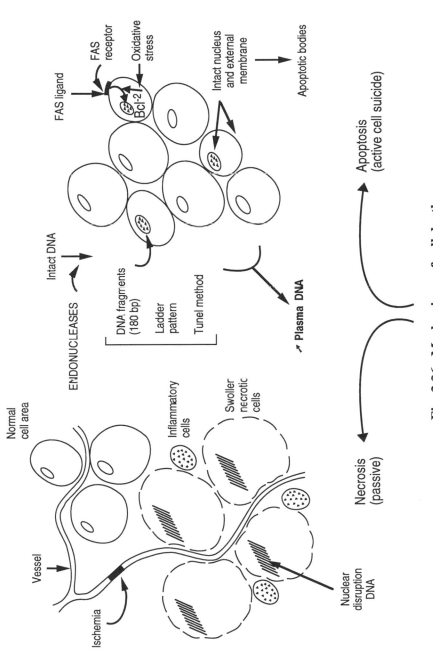

Fig. 2.26. Mechanisms of cell death

Apoptosis qualifies a genetically programed cell death due to the activation of an endogenous endonuclease. In contrast to necrosis, apoptosis is commonly viewed by its requirement for *de novo* gene expression. Consequently, apoptosis is sensitive to mRNA or protein synthesis inhibitors. The most characteristic aspect of apoptosis is DNA fragmentation, which can be histologically detected using the TUNEL technique and produces the characteristic "ladder" when size-fractionated by electrophoresis. Apoptosis is also associated with the expression of a number of regulatory genes commonly used as markers of apoptosis, including *Bcl2*, an antiapoptotic proto-oncogene, *Fas*, a proapoptotic gene, as well as others. There ais compelling evidence in support of reactive oxygen species (including superoxide and hydrogen peroxide) apoptosis occurring not only during hypoxia or ischemia but also after overstretch and NO apoptosis. During cardiac development the rate of DNA degradation diminished and is inversely related to *Bcl-2* levels [Kajstura et al. 1996].

This topic is becoming very popular in cardiology [Bing 1994] because apoptosis is rather easy to be identified. Pharmacological and pathophysiological levels of angiotensin II and catecholamines produce myocyte necrosis and coronary artery damage. Angiotensin II directly antagonized nitric oxide (NO) donor-induced apoptosis.

3

CARDIAC AND VASCULAR REMODELLING

Remodelling qualifies changes that result in the rearrangement of normally existing structures. Although remodelling does not necessarily define a pathological condition, myocardial remodelling usually results in a diseased state. The above definition eliminates gestational and developmental aspects. Remodelling concerns the two components of the cardiovascular system. The structure of both the myocardium and the vessels, including the coronary vessels, is indeed able to change under the influence of external factors, such as ischemia and mechanical overload.

Cardiac and vascular hypertrophy is not per se a disease but is the physiological adaptation of the heart to a disease, and the causal disease is coronary insufficiency and/or arterial hypertension. Cardiac remodelling commonly refers to structural rearrangements that follow myocardial infarction. Nevertheless, the definition is commonly extended to any type of cardiac hypertrophy (CH). From a biological point of view, remodelling results from a combination of the adaptational process plus two to three additional factors - namely, fibrosis, cell death, and possibly the specific phenotypic modifications of myocytes that are due to the trophic effects of circulating hormones and peptides. Cardiac failure (CF) indicates the limits of the mechanical adaptation and is aggravated, or caused, by these additional factors. The senescent heart, in the absence of any cardiovascular disease is mainly, while not solely, an overloaded heart. The overload results from the enhanced characteristic impedance of the large vessels that is the basic characteristic of the senescent vessels.

172

CARDIAC HYPERTROPHY AND FAILURE

Ventricular adaptation, and dysadaptation, is a species-specific process because the regulation of contraction differs from one animal species to the other and also because the causes of CH could differ according to the species [Swynghedauw 1990]. The biological mechanisms responsible for cardiac remodelling in humans are now better known because of cardiac transplantations which allows a direct access to cardiac tissue in human [Hasenfuss et al. 1992].

From an anatomical point of view, early ventricular remodelling following coronary occlusion is dominated by the process of infarct expansion, which is an acute dilation of the infarction area that cannot be explained by additional myocardial necrosis. Infarct expansion is caused by death and slippage of the myocytes.

Chronic ventricular remodelling includes infarct expansion of akinetic-dyskinetic segments, volume-overload hypertrophy of noninfarcted segments, and a progressive diminution of distensibility due to myocardial fibrosis. Systolic ejection decreases in propotion to the degree of remodelling.

From a biological point of view, cardiac remodelling is a complex phenomenon that results from changes in both the cardiocytes and the interstitial tissue.

Phenotypic changes in cardiocytes

In response to mechanical stimuli, both the myocardial and the vascular myocytes adapt to increased workloads through changes in gene expression that more or less reproduce the fetal programme (Table 3. 1).

Table 3. 1. Permanent changes in gene expression in compensatory cardiac hypertrophy in rat. (from Moalic et al. 1993; Swynghedauw et al. 1994).

Sarcomere

$\Downarrow$ myosin ATPase specific activity

Myosin heavy chains become $\beta\beta$

Atrial (fetal) myosin light chain expression.

No changes in thin filament

External membrane proteins

Shift from α2- to α3-subunit in Na^+, K^+-ATPase

= calcium channels

$\Uparrow$ Na^+/Ca^{2+} exchanger

$\Uparrow$ action potential duration

$\Downarrow$ I_{to}

$\Downarrow$ β1-adrenergic and muscarinic (M2) receptors

$\Uparrow$ angiotensin II receptors 1 and 2

= adenosine receptors

Sarcoplasmic reticulum proteins

$\Downarrow$ ryanodine receptors

$\Downarrow$ Ca^{2+} ATPase

$\Downarrow$ phospholamban

Energy Metabolism

$\Downarrow$ myoglobin

$\Uparrow$ mitochondrial proteins (DNA loops)

Shift to creatine kinase B

Shift to lactate deshydrogenase MM

Metabolic shift to anaerobic

Note: $\Downarrow$ decreased, $\Uparrow$ enhanced, = unchanged

Such an endogenous genetic programme is commonly associated with several other programmes resulting from complex and variable interactions between genetic and environmental factors, hormones, neurotransmitters, and peptides.

The process of adaptation

Biological adaptation is a general process by which an organ or organism changes its genetic expression and express a new genetic programme in response to new environmental requirements that unbalance its thermodynamic status. This is a necessity, and if the modifications do not result in a new and improved thermodynamic status, the organ or organism simply does not survive (and reproduce), and there is consequently no adaptation. There is no finalism in this basic process; the finalism is in fact defined *a posteriori*.

The main characteristic of biological adaptation to cardiac overload is that the thermodynamic status of the heart becomes adapted to new environmental requirements. Mechanical overload on the skeletal muscle immediately reduces the instantaneous shortening velocity by simply bringing into play the mechanical properties of the myofiber (Figure 3. 1). The load is greater; therefore, the fiber contracts more slowly which results in an immediate decrease in the economy of the system (that is the amount of developed tension per mole of ATP burnt), since the muscle fiber, as a car, is adapted to have an optimal economy for a given velocity. The process is not finalist and proceeds by trial and error, using the preexisting genetic programme, which in the heart is the fetal program. By definition there are modifications in gene expression that are beneficial, whereas others are either detrimental or even useless, and finally the modifications in the genetic expression are not limited to one gene but concerns all the cell components.

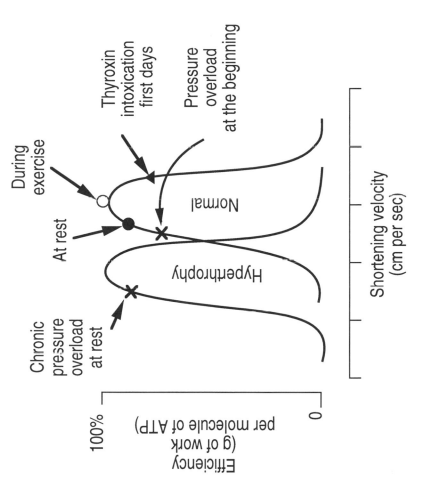

Fig. 3.1. Efficiency as a trigger for adaptation

176

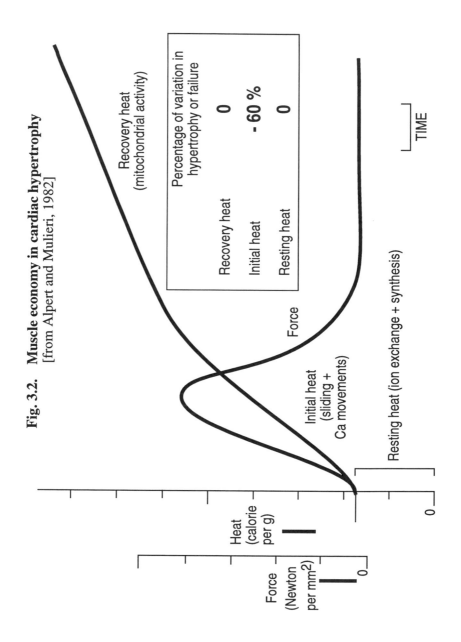

Fig. 3.2. Muscle economy in cardiac hypertrophy
[from Alpert and Mulieri, 1982]

Recovery heat (mitochondrial activity)

Percentage of variation in hypertrophy or failure	
Recovery heat	0
Initial heat	-60 %
Resting heat	0

Force

Initial heat (sliding + Ca movements)

Resting heat (ion exchange + synthesis)

TIME

Heat (calorie per g)

Force (Newton per mm²)

0

0

The change in genetic expression will allow the heart to obtain a lower Vmax and to recover a normal economy. By comparison, for a car, when we are permanently obliged to go slower and maintain a normal economy, we have to change the motor. The change in gene expression has not been directed toward this finality by a magic finger; in fact, facing this new situation the genome simply uses another programme. There are not many available, and the program used in the heart is most likely to be the fetal one.

Table 3. 2. Economy of the hypertrophied heart. Data are recalculated from Alpert and Mulieri [1982 and 1992] and expressed in percentage of control.

Degree of hypertrophy	45%*
Resulting increase in force	17%*
Resting heat (synthesis, ionic movements)	Unchanged
Heat produced by mechanical activity	- 58%*
Heat produced by mitochondria	Unchanged
Economy of the system	102%

* The difference is significant.

Cardiac hypertrophy

The increase in cardiac mass is the most easily detectable adaptational factor triggered by mechanical overload. Cardiac hypertrophy adapts the heart to the new working conditions by both multiplying the contractile units and reducing the wall stress according to the Laplace law.

A considerable amount of work using radioactive amino acid labelling was performed on this topic before the arrival of molecular biological techniques. Extensive reviews were previously published on the topic. In brief, the activation of protein synthesis is a rapid and rather homogeneous phenomena. Total protein, myosin, but not myoglobin and collagen synthesis were activated after 3 h of increased aortic pressure. P.Y. Hatt et al. [1965] was able to evidence polysomes into the myocardium 30 minutes after the imposition of an acute overload. Following imposition of a pressure overload, as aortic stenosis, radioactive labelling of total proteins or myosin remains unchanged for one or 2 days, peaks at 5 to 6 days, and returns to control values within 2 to 3 weeks. The accumulation of total proteins or myosin is due to an increased rate of synthesis. Nevertheless, the rate of degradation is augmented in parallel. Such a paradoxical wasting effect is a general feature in protein metabolism [Moalic et al. 1984]. Molecular biological techniques using global approaches such as hybridization curves to evaluate mRNA complexity were unable to detect major differences between normal and hypertrophied hearts [de la Bastie et al. 1987]. Different results were in fact obtained later on using more sophisticated techniques, such as differential display and specific hybridization procedures, and are detailed below.

Energetics
Several changes in genetic expression allow the heart to recover a normal economy. According to Laplace's law, cardiac hypertrophy will normalize the wall stress. Simultaneously, qualitative changes will allow the myocardial fiber to contract more slowly and to recover a normal economy by having a lower maximum shortening velocity (V_{max}) and by using a different force/velocity curve. To quantify this economy, it is necessary to measure the energy flux by measuring ATP or oxygen consumption or heat production (Figure 3. 2). The heart, as any other muscle, is using energy for several purposes. The fundamental process of adaptation that occurs both in human and in experimental models includes a slowing of V_{max} with a diminution of the heat produced per g of active tension during contraction: both the resting and recovery heats remain unchanged. Special experimental

protocols allow the partitioning of heat produced by the sliding process, from heat produced by the movements of calcium and the activity of the different calcium pumps. Both systems function more economically in cardiac hypertrophy and in end-stage cardiac failure in humans [Alpert and Mulieri 1982, Alpert et al. 1992, Hasenfuss et al. 1992] (Table 3. 2).

In conclusion: (1) the reduction in Vmax is the main basic process responsible for myocardial adaptation to mechanical overload, and thermodynamic data suggest that this reduction is due to a decreased recruitment of myosin cross-bridges. (2) In sharp contrast with the current bedside opinion, the diminution of Vmax has a beneficial effect, since it allows the cardiac myofiber to produce energy at a normal energy cost. Nevertheless, at the organ level, the diminution of Vmax is also the first step of CF. (3) Perturbed energy metabolism is an unlikely candidate for the cause of CF since the "recovery heat" remains unchanged. Hence, investigations concerning the adaptational process have been mainly focusing on energy utilization rather than energy production. (4) Such modifications already exist in compensated CH and also exist both in the experimental models and in the clinical situation.

Energy metabolism

Whether CF is caused by a defect in energy production or a deficit in energy utilization is an continuing debate [Meerson 1969]. Of course, it is easy to oppose CF due to an acute anoxia and CF due to a massive loss in contractile tissue caused by myocardial infarction, nevertheless these are rare situations. In fact the real problem is to know whether, during the compensatory stage, modifications in mitochondria or anaerobic energy pathways could account for further impairment of myocardial function or whether, conversely, CF could be more easily explained by a deficit in either the contractile protein or the calcium movements.

Global studies on energy metabolism favour the second hypothesis. Myocardial oxygen, substrate uptake, and ATP content are normal in CF, even in humans. One of the most convincing experiments was from Peter Pool et al. [1968]. Pool et al. showed that freshly isolated papillary muscle from a failing cat heart had both reduced shortening velocity and a low creatine phosphate content. Nevertheless, when the muscles were left in an oxygenated bath for half an hour, they recover normal high-energy phosphate stores even though the contractile velocity remained hampered.

A pronounced reduction in myocardial myoglobin protein has been well documented in various models of CF in humans, and such a reduction could be considered as one of the energy-saving adaptations [O'Brien et al. 1995]. In compensated CH, mitochondria adapt to the new situation by increasing their number and decreasing their size [Hatt et al. 1970]. The mitochondrial mass increases by activation of mitochondrial DNA replication and by removal of the block in the conversion of DNA D-loops to other intermediates, and *in vitro* studies showed normal or even improved mitochondrial oxygen function and coupling. One of the rare detailed studies on cardiac metabolism in the CH demonstrates an increased glucose utilization and a pronounced enhancement in the activity of glycolysis together with a diminished activity of enzymes responsible for ketone body metabolism [Taegmeyer and Overturf 1988]. Failure induces a depression in mitochondrial function and modifications in several of the mitochondrial enzymes including malate and glutamate deshydrogenase [Peters et al. 1977]. To conclude, there is no doubt that CH is associated with a shift from aerobic to anaerobic metabolism.

Ion currents

The increased QT interval duration on ECG and action potential on isolated cardiomyocytes are well-documented characteristics of the hypertrophied heart [Hart 1994; Swynghedauw and Coraboeuf 1994; Assayag et al. 1997]

(Table 3. 3). Acquired modifications of the repolarization time are likely to reflect the adaptational response and to be caused by one or several change in ion currents [Assayag et al. 1997; Swynghedauw et al. 1997] (see below "Long QT syndrome" for the inherited alterations of the QT interval). (1) The major defect in mechanical overload is a pronounced depression of the early transient outward K^+ current, I_{to}, after normalization to cell surface area [Coulombe et al. 1994]. This modification reflects changes in the genetic expression of the corresponding K^+ channels gene. The expression of the corresponding Kv clones, which encode I_{to}, are indeed decreased by more than 50%, suggesting that the diminution of the corresponding K^+ current, and the corresponding lengthening of both action potential and QT, are transcriptionally regulated and participate in the adaptational process [Gidh-Jain et al. 1996]. Gene transfer using a prototype of the voltage-dependent class of K^+ channels is able to correct such a defect. (2) The current density and the total number of calcium channels remain unchanged; nevertheless, this is accompanied by isoform modifications. During CF, the density of the calcium channels could be different, which has been attributed to a direct effect of plasma catecholamines. (3) Sodium-calcium exchange creates an inward depolarizing current. There are arguments suggesting that such a current is prolonged as a consequence of the prolongation of the calcium transient. (4) Two currents (I_f, I_{CaT}) and the $\alpha 3$-isoform of the (Na^+, K^+) ATPase, which all are specific for the sinus node, have been found in overloaded ventricles, suggesting that the ventricles are able to acquire some degree of automaticity. (5) There are evidence of complex rearrangements of connexin distribution in CH with a shift from connexin 43 to connexin 40, which may be the molecular substrate for explaining the increased susceptibility of the hypertrophied heart to ischemia.

Table 3. 3. Ion current and channels in cardiac hypertrophy and cardiac failure. Human usually means CF, experimental models usually mean compensated CH.

	Human	Experimental models
ECG		
QT interval)	⇑	⇑
Electrophysiology		
Cell membrane capacitance	⇑	⇑
Action potential duration	⇑	⇑
Resting potential	=	=
Intracellular calcium transient		
Duration	⇓	⇑
Peak	⇓	=
Resting current	⇑	⇓
Patch-clamp studies (Normalized currents)		
Outward K^+ currents		
I_{to}	⇓	⇓
I_{ks}	=	⇓
I_{k1}	⇓	?
Ik_{ATP}	⇓	?
Inward currents		
I_{Na}	=	?
I_{CaL}	⇓	=
$I_{Na\text{-}Ca}$	?	?
Pacemaker like currents		
I_{CaT}	?	Present
I_f	?	Present

Ion channels (protein and mRNA)

K^+ channel subunit mRNA and protein

Kv 4.2	⇓	?
Kv 1.4 and *2.1*	⇓	?

Note: ⇓ decreased, ⇑ enhanced, = unchanged, ? not documented

Control of intracellular pH ([pH_i])

Pressure overload in rabbit increases the Na^+-H^+ antiporter isoform NHE-1 mRNA by two fold by the third day after imposition of the load. The same type of activation has been observed in response to ischemia. In contrast, the activity of the exchanger is reduced in the diabetic heart in response to the alterations of intracellular calcium.

Calcium regulating proteins

An altered calcium uptake of SR and a decreased concentration of both the SR calcium ATPase and phospholamban in CH and CF are now well documented (Figure 3. 3). Todate the diminished expression of SERCA 2a, the gene encoding the cardiac isoform of the enzyme, is considered to be one of the best markers of chronic cardiac overload (Table 3. 1) [de la Bastie et al. 1990; Lompré et al. 1991]. The reduction in the concentration of the enzyme is progressive and linked to the progression of CH. Adenovirus-mediated expression of a SERCA 2 transgene can reconstitute endogenous SERCA levels and activity obtained in cultured neonatal cardiocytes treated with phorbol-12-myristate-13-acetate. It is then conceivable to correct the above SERCA deficit using gene transfer technology.

Two forms of intracellular calcium-release channels are expressed in the heart. The situation for the ryanodine receptors is rather complicated. In compensated CH, the ryanodine receptor binding site density is reduced and parallels the Ca^{2+}-ATPase. In end-stage CF in humans several articles, including one from our laboratory [Sainte-Beuve et al. 1997] found a decreased mRNA content and an unchanged protein level. In addition, binding studies using radioactive ryanodine revealed a twofold increase in the number of high-affinity sites, suggesting that during CF additional regulatory factors affect the ryanodine binding properties.

Calcium entry from the extracellular space is normal [Scamps et al. 1990], except in end-stage failure. Calcium output is mainly regulated by a functional duo composed of the Na^+/Ca^{2+} exchanger and the (Na^+, K^+)-ATPase (Fig. 2. 1). Both are modified in CH, suggesting that calcium homeostasis may be unbalanced at this level. Modifications in the sodium pump are species-specific. In the rat the specific activity is unchanged and there are several modifications reflecting an isoenzymic shift of the α-subunit from the adult form ($\alpha2$) to the fetal form ($\alpha3$). In rat, $\alpha3$ has a much lower affinity for sodium than $\alpha2$, and this shift finally results in a lower affinity of the overall enzyme for sodium [Lelièvre et al. 1986; Charlemagne et al. 1986; 1994]. The situation is different in humans, where the activity of the ATPase is reduced and is less sensitive to sodium. Molecular biological studies have found a shift from the $\alpha1$ to the $\alpha3$ isoform. Since the human heart possesses an $\alpha1$-subunit with a low affinity for sodium, one can conclude that in humans, as in rats, the final result is a diminution of the affinity of sodium for the enzyme and a slight accumulation of sodium below the membrane surface.

The activity of the Na^+/Ca^{2+} exchanger has been a controversial issue [Hanf et al. 1988; Studer et al. 1994]. It is now been generally accepted that the molecular density of the Na^+/Ca^{2+} exchanger is increased during both compensatory hypertrophy and in end-stage cardiac failure in humans [Studer et al. 1994]. The Na^+/Ca^{2+} exchanger is an electrogenic transporter that generates a current. The prolongation of the calcium transient will lengthen the I_{Na-Ca}, and at present it is thought that the activity of the exchanger is both lengthened and attenuated by the slightest increase in intracellular sodium.

Cardiac receptors

Numerous changes in the expression of most of the known myocardial receptors have been reported (Table 3. 1). They are likey to reflect both an adaptation to the mechanical stress (- that is a heterologous regulation), and additional homologous regulations in response to changes in the plasma levels of the corresponding agonists.

Following the pioneer studies of M. Bristow [Bristow et al. 1982], the cardiac *β-adrenergic receptors* have been extensively investigated [Brodde 1991], and two situations have to be clearly separated. (1) Studies on compensated CH have shown that, despite normal plasma levels and depressed myocardial catecholamine content, the β-adrenergic receptor density and its mRNA are decreased by 30%, suggesting a heterologous downregulation; the corresponding gene is not activated by mechanical stress; the changes in receptor density are pretranslationnally regulated [Mansier et al. 1993]. (2) In CF, the elevated circulating catecholamine levels induces a homologous down-regulation that induces an additional decrease in the receptor density. *Muscarinic receptors* and mRNAs are also down-regulated in CCH [Mansier et al. 1993], and, at least in the rat, the muscarinic/b1-adrenergic receptor ratio remains unchanged. One of the most prominent features of CF, which has been confirmed by several laboratories, is the existence of a 75% increase in G_{ia-2}. Such an alteration could account for the discrepancies between changes in adrenoceptor density and the adenylate-cyclase stimulating effects of agonists. The increased level of this particular G subunit in cardiac failure is most likely to be caused by elevated levels of plasma catecholamines [Eschenhagen et al. 1992].

The decreased β1-adrenergic receptor density protects the heart against acute stress and, in CH, participates in the overall process of cardiac

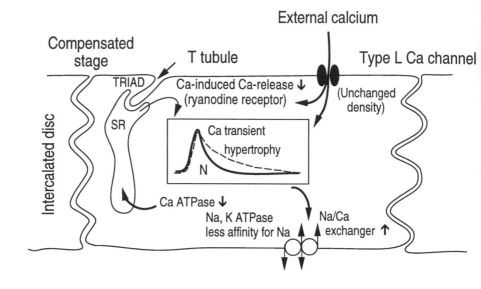

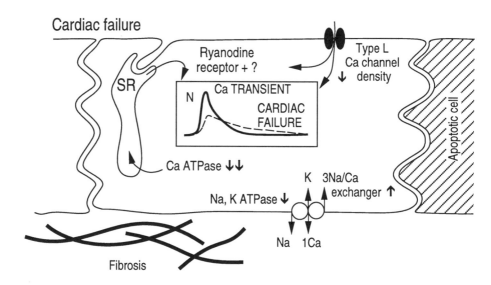

Fig. 3.3. **Membrane composition during compensated
CH and cardiac failure**

adaptation by attenuating the inotropic effects of catecholamines (Figure 3. 3). As such, noninduction of the genes encoding this system has the same significance as noninduction of the SR Ca^{2+} ATPase.

Angiotensin II receptors (ATR) are expressed at a rather low density in the heart, as compared to the β-adrenergic receptors. Reactive hypertrophy after myocardial infarction is accompanied by a 2- to 4-fold increase in ATR1A and ATR2 density which parallels the depression in the velocity of myocyte shortening and is transcriptionally regulated. Such an augmentation occurs soon after acute infarction in the zone of acute ischemia and then remains located in the scar tissue and noninfarcted fibrotic area [Nio et al. 1995]. In several reports, except 2, models of compensated CH results in substantial increases in ventricular ATR receptors with an unchanged AT1/AT2 receptor ratio. CF is accompanied by a pronounced loss of AT1R [Regitz-Zagrosck et al. 1995], not ATR2. The drop in AT1R density is correlated with the decrease in β1-adrenergic density, suggesting that the 2 phenomena have a common origin and may be related to the increased plasma levels of the corresponding agonists [Asano et al. 1997].

Contractile proteins

In phylogeny when different muscles from various species are compared, a good correlation has been found between myosin ATPase - that is the type of *MHC isoform,* including "superactivated" ATPase and Vmax, in various conditions including mechanical overload, thyroxin intoxication and the right to left ventricles differences [Swynghedauw 1986]. In response to chronic mechanical overload, myocyte genes from various striated muscles respond in the same way whatever the muscle type - that is atria, ventricular, or fast skeletal muscle. The response includes an inhibition of the expression of those genes coding for fast MHC, which differ in the heart (α-MHC), in the skeletal muscle (MHCf), and in an activation of a unique gene (β-MHC), in all three muscles. Such harmonious and complex regulations require a common mechanism for the 2 muscles and for the 3 genes - α-MHC, MHC_f, and β-MHC. The regulation is mostly, if not entirely, transcriptional [Lompré et al. 1984].

The first evidence of qualitative (and reversible) changes in the molecular structure of the overloaded heart was made in our laboratory and consists in a MHC shift observed in the overloaded rat ventricle [Lompré et al. 1979]. Subsequently similar modifications were confirmed by numerous groups in different models of cardiac overload in rats and mice. In the heart, these isomyosin changes depend on both animal species and muscle type (Table 3. 1. In the rat ventricle the αα-isoform is predominant; in contrast, the normal human ventricle is entirely composed of the slow MHC isoform ββ. In the rat ventricle, cardiac overload rapidly induces a shift from the αα to the ββ-MHC isoform [Lompré et al. 1979], which correlates with the shortening velocity [Schwartz et al. 1981]. The increased amount of β-MHC mRNA precedes the protein changes, which demonstrates that the level of the regulation is pretranslational. By day 2 to 3 after aortic banding, β-MHC mRNA was hardly detectable and was mainly restricted to the inner part of the left ventricle and around the coronary arteries of both ventricles. This suggests that the signal originates from the hemodynamic changes [Schiaffino et al. 1989]. In humans, as well as in several other mammalian species, such a shift occurs but is of minor importance since the human ventricle is already composed almost entirely of the ββ-MHC [Leclercq et al. 1976; Mercadier et al. 1987; Clapier-Ventura et al. 1988]. Myosin ATPase isolated from human ventricles is unmodified by mechanical overload, even when it is fully activated by cross-linking with actin [Lauer et al. 1989].

In every mammalian species so far studied, normal atrial muscle shortens faster than the ventricle. Consequently, the atrial content of the αα-MHC chain isoform is always much higher than that of the ββ-isoform. Atrial overload is accompanied by a decreased content in αα-MHC which parallels the echocardiographically determined atrial size [Mercadier et al.

1987]. Hence, in humans, changes in the expression of genes encoding contractile proteins account for the enhanced contractility of atria, which compensates for the depressed early ventricular filling and, in part, the modifications of both ventricular contractility and active relaxation.

The overloaded human atria possesses, in addition to their normal content of specific atrial light chains, the ventricular *MlC subtypes*, MlC_{1v}, and $MPlC_{2v}$. In addition, in various forms of human cardiomyopathies, the ventricles become enriched in the embryonic MlC isoform, MlC_{emb} (which is also, in fact, the MlC expressed in the atria) in proportion to the degree of ventricular wall stress and that after valve replacement the amount of MlC_{1a} returns to a normal level [Hirzel et al. 1985; Sütsch et al. 1992].

Thin filament proteins are not thought to be modified during chronic overload. The transient expression of the skeletal mRNA isoform that has been reported after aortic banding can have a physiological significance. Studies with BALB/c mice, which express abnormally high levels of α-skeletal actin in the heart showed indeed that such increased levels of the skeletal isoform were significantly correlated with this increased contractility.

There are no convincing experiments in favor of a deficit of the sensitivity of the contractile apparatus to calcium as a mechanism to explain CF. Investigations performed in various models using chemically skinned fibers showed enhanced maximum calcium activated force, but unchanged calcium sensitivity occurred in the overloaded ventricles, not in atria [Clapier-Ventura et al. 1988].

Cardiac cycle

Several converging reports have demonstrated in compensated CH a lengthening of the calcium transient that parallels the increased action potential duration in both clinical and experimental settings [Gwathmey et al. 1987; 1990]. More controversial results have been reported in CF with a significantly depressed peak $(Ca^{2+})_i$ and a slowing of the rate of diastolic calcium decay.

The most important physiological determinant of the calcium transient (and isometric twitch tension) is the stimulation frequency. There are no studies of this sort dealing with compensated CH, and very few studies have even addressed this question in CF [Pieske et al. 1995]. The work of Pieske et al. [1995] was performed at the physiological temperature of 37°C and over the whole physiological frequency range of 15 to 180 min^{-1}. He showed that at low stimulation frequency the peak of $(Ca^{2+})_i$ was unchanged in muscle strips from a failing human heart. When the stimulation frequency was increased to 120 min^{-1}, both the peak aequorin light and isometric tension increased in strips from normal hearts. In contrast, the failing heart showed a decrease in both of these two parameters.

Myocyte loss and abnormalities in ECM components are unlikely to be solely responsible for the depression of the depressed ventricular function in CF and are associated with an impairment of the contractile properties of individual cardiocytes.

Excitation-contraction coupling (ECC)

The normal myocardial ECC includes a voltage-dependent gating of calcium channels, which results in a local increased $(Ca^{2+})_i$. Further on, a calcium-induced calcium-release occurs through the ryanodine receptors. This phenomenon is facilitated by the close proximity of the sarcolemmal calcium channels and ryanodine receptors in the dyads and can be directly observed in the confocal microscope as calcium sparks. The released calcium can then activate contraction, and tension develops commensuratly with the peak of the calcium transient.

A direct approach is to evaluate the ability of I_{CaL} to provoke calcium release by measuring the number of calcium sparks and integrating

I_{CaL} during a voltage-clamp pulse [Gomez et al. 1997]. The probability of evoking calcium sparks is markedly reduced in experimental models of both compensated and decompensated cardiac hypertrophy at all potentials, while I_{CaL} density and voltage dependence remained unchanged. The proposed explanation for such an uncoupling was based on ultrastructural data suggesting that the distance between the calcium channels and SR structures is enhanced.

Calcium homeostasis

Several experiments had provided direct and indirect evidence that the ability of the hypertrophied cardiac myocyte to buffer any changes in $(Ca^{2+})_i$ is reduced (Fig. 3. 3) [Brutsaert 1989]. (1) Stepwise increases in the calcium concentration of a perfusate of an isolated heart preparation resulted in ventricular fibrillation and spontaneous calcium oscillations at a calcium concentration above 10 mM. Such a threshold is around 6 to 8 mM in CII. (2) The normal isolated rat heart becomes stiffer when perfused for 5 to 10 minutes in anoxic conditions. This phenomenon is exaggerated in CH [Callens-ElAmrani et al. 1992]. (3) Several experimental studies have demonstrated a predisposition of CH to ventricular arrhythmias [Assayag et al. 1997 a].

The hypothesis which, for the moment, best fits the data is the following (Fig. 3. 3). (1) During the compensatory stage the diastolic $(Ca^{2+})_i$ is normal but the transient is prolonged to allow the heart to contract more slowly and to maintain its normal economy, as explained above (Fig. 3. 2). Nevertheless, the cell is incapable of controlling any abnormal influx of calcium, due, for example, to anoxia, ischemia, inotropic agents, or various stresses. The activity of the SR is slowed down, and, at the external membrane level, the calcium influx increases in proportion to the degree of cardiac hypertrophy. Nevertheless, the prolongation of the calcium transient lengthens I_{Na-Ca}. Simultaneously, calcium release through the exchanger is hampered. (2) During CF, there is a secretion of several hormones or peptides, including catecholamines, angiotensin II, and endothelin, all of which have a trophic effect. The peak of the calcium transient is now decreased, and the myocardial phenotype is diffrent as compared to compensated CH. These modifications may vary depending on the predominant additional factor. Convincing data have shown a diminution of the calcium channels density that may aggravate the disturbances in calcium homeostasis. At the level of the SR unexplained modifications occur in the ryanodine receptor.

Cardiac autocrine functions

There is evidence that the first two endocrine secretions of the heart - namely, ANF and angiotensin II - are activated during CH, and that catecholamine cardiac stores are depleted.

The ANF is normally expressed only in the atria. ANF expression and secretion are activated in overloaded atria and induced in overloaded ventricles [Mercadier et al. 1989]. The ventricular expression of ANF, and of other natriuretic peptides (brain and C-type natriuretic peptides), is actually considered to be the best biological marker of ventricular overload. ANF interacts with particulate guanylate cyclase in target cells to produce cGMP both *in vivo* and *in vitro*. As a consequence, urinary cGMP is considered as an easily measurable humoral second messenger of the ANF system [Michel et al. 1990]. A marked overexpression of the brain form seems a special feature of hypertrophic obstructive cardiomyopathy.

A major peripheral factor of adaptation to changes in hemodynamic conditions occurring during CF is the activation of the circulating RAS and aldosterone production, which both contribute to maintain a normal arterial pressure by increasing the peripheral resistance's and plasma volume. The myocardial RAS is activated by mechanical stretch and in any type of mechanical overload.

Endothelin-1 and prepro-endothelin-1 mRNA were significantly increased in several experimental models of CF. Such an upregulation correlates with the left ventricular end-diastolic pressure. In humans, the elevation of plasma endothelin-1 became significant in patients with moderate CF (NYHA classes III and IV). Nevertheless, there is, for the moment, no clear evidence of a stimulation of the myocardial production of the peptide in the failing human heart.

Basal circulating NO levels nearly double in idiopathic dilated cardiomyopathy. iNOS mRNA and protein are not present in the normal human heart, but they are coexpressed with ANF in the myocardium of patients with CF independent of the cause, which raises the possibility that autocrine and paracrine actions of iNOS may be of physiopathological importance.

Plasma catecholamines increase in proportion to the severity of CF as a consequence of the hemodynamic deficit. Norepinephrine stores are depleted in every kind of decompensated cardiac hypertrophy as initially shown by Chidsey et al. [1966]. Such a depletion is under local rather than systemic control.

An increasing body of evidences supports the existence of paracrine and autocrine growth pathways in the myocardium. Nevertheless, it is, for the moment impossible to decide whether such an activation has really functional consequences. Tumor necrosis factor-α (TNF-α) is a proinflammatory cytokine that has a cytolytic effect and produces negative inotropic effects. The plasma level of both TNF-α and interleukin-6 is normal in patients with compensated CH and enhanced in advanced congestive CF.

Cytoskeleton

There are many lines of evidence that suggest that there is an early transient reorganization of the microtubular network and an activated expression of β-

actin 2 to 4 days after mechanical overload [Rappaport and Samuel 1988]. Permanent changes in the microtubules were reported more recently. Both the microtubular network and tubulin concentration were indeed augmented in pressure-overloaded cat ventricles. Volume overload showed no changes. It has been proposed that the microtubule component of the cytoskeleton imposes a resistive intracellular load on sarcomere shortening and, formed in excess, impedes sarcomere motion [Tsutsui et al. 1993].

Other cytoskeletal proteins could also play a role in maintaining a certain degree of cardiocyte stiffness. Titin protein expression is enhanced both in experimental decompensated CH and in the failing human heart and may participate in the impairment of contractility. Desmin, which forms intermediate filaments, is equally augmented and disorderly arranged. The amount of vinculin present in the cardiocytes is increased in dilated cardiomyopathy. Changes in these cytoskeleton components could compensate for the loss in contractile material, thereby maintaining the cell shape [Schaper and Speiser 1992].

Phenotypic changes in ECM

Type of fibrosis
Collagen mass, and not collagen concentration, increases in parallel with CH and participates in the rpocess of adaptation. Fibrosis is an increased concentration in collagen and has different origins. Fibrosis is not directly induced by stretch or mechanical overload and did not participate in the adaptational process [Weber and Brilla 1991; Weber et al. 1993; Assayag et al. 1997a]. Fibrosis enhances myocardial stiffness because collagen I is a very rigid protein (the tensile strength of collagen fiber approaches that of steel), generates arrhythmias because fibrosis creates myocardial electrical heterogeinity and reentry, and hampers systolic ejection by rendering the myocardium heterogeneous. It is common to distinguish between reparative

and reactive fibrosis. Reparative fibrosis occurs as a reaction to a loss of myocardial material due to cell death and is mainly interstitial. In contrast, reactive fibrosis is observed as a reaction to inflammation and is primarily perivascular. During cardiac remodelling reactive and reparative fibrosis usually coexist. Fibrosis is multifactorial and caused by myocardial ischemia or hypoxia, senescence, inflammatory processes, diabetes or several hormones or vasoactive peptides [Weber and Brilla 1991; Weber et al. 1993; Assayag et al. 1997].

Causes of fibrosis

The woundhealing response of the myocardium after infarction involves both the infarcted area and the noninfarcted ventricle. Reparative fibrosis is organized as a scar and is surrounded by reactive fibrosis in the noninfarcted area and compensatory myocyte hypertrophy. Ischemia is first associated with inflammatory cells, which produces transforming-growth factor-β1 (TGF-β1). TGF-β1 transforms fibroblasts into myofibroblasts that produce various forms of collagenases. The initial modifications of the ECM are collagen degradation and desorganization and are responsiblefor infarct expansion and myocyte slippage. Constituted scar is formed several weeks after infarction and is accompanied by development of fibrosis in the noninfarcted area of the left ventricle. The mechanism responsible for fibrogenesis in such areas is still debatable and may involve diffusion through the interstitial space of signals that appear in the ischemic area [Michel et al. 1990; Weber et al. 1993].

Angiotensin II is fibrogenic because angiotensin II acts both as a growth factor and a potent vasoconstrictor. Perfusion with nonhypotensive dosis of the peptide generates fibrosis. Fibrosis is then delayed and not associated with preceeding necrosis and may implicate coronary vascular hyperpermeability. There is also evidence based on experiments performed on isolated fibroblasts that angiotensin II can directly activate collagen synthesis [Brilla et al. 1990]. Angiotensin II and endothelin-1 may act synergistically to create fibrosis.

Aldosterone infusion to uninephrectomized rats plus a high-salt diet induces perivascular and interstitial fibrosis in the absence of any activation of the RAS in the two ventricles, in the atria, and around the big vessels, suggesting a diffuse process that is not linked to the mechanical overload [Brilla et al. 1990; Robert et al. 1994; 1997]. The aldosterone-induced fibrosis is both   and is accompanied by necrosis. It is likely to be pretranslationally regulated [Robert et al. 1994] and to have multiple origins. Fibrosis is not caused by a reduced collagenase activities and is accompanied by an upregulation of ATR. Aldosterone-induced cardiac fibrosis is prevented by spironoactone and losartan suggesting that ATR could be responsible for the fibrosis.

Daily injection of isoprenaline in rats for 10 days generates subendocardial myocyte death and stable reparative fibrosis whithout perivascular fibrosis in the noninvolved areas. Subendocardial fibrillar collagen encircles endocardial muscle fibers, which atrophy, and this leads to reduced active tension.

Pressure overload is frequently associated with fibrosis. Nevertheless, there are models of pressure overload with normal collagen concentration, and it was proposed that, in fact, fibrosis, which is observed in this condition, is caused by associated factors linked to arterial hypertension like ischemia, senescence, diabetes, and plasma hormones or peptides (as in renovascular hypertension) [Weber et al. 1993]. Rather ancient morphometric autopsy studies in humans have constantly evidenced in hypertensive cardiopathy an increased collagen volume fraction with interstitial and perivascular fibrosis and microscopic scarring [reviewed in Weber and Brilla 1991; Schaper and Speiser 1992]. Clinical quantitation of ventricular fibrosis is now possible by serum procollagen peptide measurements. Fibrosis is possibly a consequence of the reduction of coronary reserve. This hypothesis is supported by the findings of myocardial microscars in most of the models.

Fibrosis is not inevitabily linked to mechanical overload, and there are several experimental and clinical models of mechanically overloaded hearts with unchanged myocardial stiffness and collagen content. The list includes chronic volume overload, exercise training, and infrarenal aortic stenosis [Apstein et al. 1987; Brilla et al. 1990].

Other components of the ECM

It is now clearly established that fibronectin accumulation preceeds that of collagen during fibrillogenesis after aortic stenosis [Farhadian et al. 1996] and is coexpressed with TGFβ1. Laminin and type IV collagen contribute to ECM assembly in healing after myocardial infarction.

Cell death

Cell death is an important determinant of CF as it causes loss of contractile tissue, compensatory hypertrophy of myocardial cells, and reparative fibrosis. A diminution of contractile material is a prominent figure in human CF, whatever the origin. Whether or not cell death reflects only the age of the population or the high incidence of ischemia is debatable. Cell death can occur either by necrosis or apoptosis.

Ischemia

In vivo experimental and clinical investigations have confirmed *in vitro* findings, strongly suggesting that apoptosis could be, in association with necrosis, an important component of postmyocardial infarction. A careful evaluation of the respective roles of these two modes of cell death was performed by Kajstura et al. in the rat model of myocardial infarction [1996] and led to the conclusion that during the first 6 hours after coronary occlusion programed cell death is the major form of myocardial damage. Necrotic cells prevailed at later times (2 days), and a similar small number of apoptotic and necrotic cells were observed by the seventh day. Studies of myocardial samples of patients who died from acute myocardial infarction confirmed the predominance of apoptotic compared to necrotic cells.

Cardiac hypertrophy and failure

Aortic banding in rats results in compensated CH and in a wave of apoptotic cardiocytes suggesting that apoptosis is a regulatory mechanism that participates in the initiation of the hypertrophic process. A few reports have recently shown an increased number of apoptotic cardiocytes in CF. It is, for the moment, impossible to decide whether apoptosis is the cause or a consequence of CF.

Transition to cardiac failure

CF is a disease state with both abnormalities in the myocardial structure and clinical symptoms due to fluid retention. The functional nature of such a definition renders difficult the experimental approach of the transition. It is indeed difficult to quantitate tachypnea in a rat! Schematically, failure may indicate the limits of the above-defined adaptational process. Fibrosis can play a crucial role, even if the adaptational process did not reach its limits. Finally, failure can be caused by a loss of muscle. In fact, the 3 reasons are frequently associated, although at various degrees. There are no specific biological markers for CF. The search for molecular markers of the transition is, for the moment, at the beginning. In the aged SHR model the only real markers of failure are probes specific for ECM components. Other possible biological markers of the transient are the disappearance of the sensitivity to β-agonists and the apoptotic index. The markers can differ

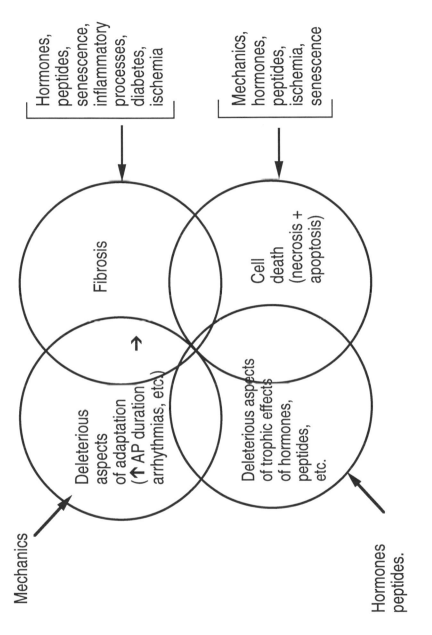

Fig. 3.4. Biological factors responsible for myocardial failure

from one model to another. In guinea pigs after aortic banding the calcium ATPase of SR were indeed only modified in CF.

Finally the following scheme can be proposed (Figure 3. 4). During cardiac remodelling, failure has a multifactorial origin and results from four differentially regulated factors, including the deleterious aspects of the process of adaptation, which are regulated by mechanics or stretch; fibrosis, which has multiple origins but did not result from mechanics; cell death due to both necrosis and apoptosis, which has multiple origins including mechanics and fibrosis; and the deleterious aspects of the trophic effects of several hormones or peptides (Figure 3. 4).

Hypertrophy of the arterial wall

Chronic arterial hypertension is one of the major causes of cardiac failure. The arterial wall responds to high blood pressure in the same way as the myocardium and hypertrophies (Tedgui et Levy 1994) in order to normalize the wall stress. Both endothelial and smooth muscle cells participate in this process: endothelial cells replicate, while smooth muscle cells either hypertrophy in the large arteries or become hyperplasic in the smaller vessels. Simultaneously, the extracellular matrix mass is modified, the elastin content remains unchanged, but collagen and fibronectin concentrations are increased. Both mechanical stress (the increased pressure and shear stress) and vasoactive peptides, such as angio II, play a major role in these phenotypic modifications.

THE SENESCENT HEART AND VESSELS

The aged heart is not only enlarged but also quite different in terms of receptor densities, a major target for drug design, and most of the observed modifications are likely to adapt the heart to the new aortic impedance.

Studies of cardiovascular senescence are far from being academic since epidemiological studies have shown that diseases of the heart are one of the major cause of mortality among the overall population and the main cause in people over 65 years of age. Therefore it is of major importance to determine the state of the heart in undiseased elderly subjects and to assess the limits of normality in aged persons.

The clinical problem is far from being simple because obviously the fundamental biological process of senescence is intimately associated with an increased incidence of arterial hypertension and atherosclerosis and also with modifications in physical activity and nutritional status, which all may seriously modify the myocardial structure. From a purely economic point of view, it is important to know if aging myocardium is similar to the myocardium of younger adults and if we can prescribe the same drugs to both groups of people. It is also important to decide if the initial screening of new therapies needs to be done in senescent animal models.

The pioneer studies in this field have been carried out by a group headed by E. Lakatta [1993] in Baltimore, who recently published an important review mostly focused on the physiological aspects of this problem. Several other review articles have also recently been published [Besse et al. 1994; Folkow and Svanborg 1993].

Anatomical and cellular data

Anatomical studies have shown that the weight of the heart regularly increases with age. This is not really a clinical hypertrophy since the heart weight/body weight ratio remains unchanged, except in people over 90, in whom a slight decrease in the ratio is observed. Clinical and experimental studies have revealed that in the aging heart, a loss of myocytes and fibrosis are associated with myocyte hypertrophy that is more significant in the left ventricle. Such a loss was only partly compensated by an enhanced myocyte volume. Cardiocyte hypertrophy is a constant finding during senescence and is much more pronounced in the left ventricle than in the right ventricle [Anversa et al. 1990].

In most mammalian species the majority of cardiac myocytes are binucleated (Rakusan and Nagai 1994). However in humans binucleation is observed only in 10% of cardiocytes In fact, the human cardiocyte becomes progressively poplyploid only with age [Adler 1975] since there is a progressive increase in both the degree of polyploid cells, the number of highly (16 n) polyploid nuclei, and the number of nucleoli.

Histochemical studies have shown an abnormal accumulation of fibrillar collagen with an increased collagen cross-linking, both around the vessels and within the interstitium. The concentration of the two main components of fibrosis - namely collagen I and fibronectin - increases during aging. By contrast, both type I and type III procollagen mRNA levels were reduced in the senescent rat heart showing that changes in myocardial collagen mRNA and protein were not synchronous, which suggests that during senescence collagen concentration is not transcriptionally regulated [Besse et al. 1994].

Table 3. 4. Senescent heart versus overloaded heart: fibrosis, arrhythmias and mechanics [from Besse et al. 1992; 1993].

	Overload	Senescence
Fibrosis	+ or 0	+++ *
Arrhythmias	+	+++ *
Mechanics		
Maximum shortening velocity	$\Downarrow$	$\Downarrow$
Maximum relengthening velocity	$\Downarrow$	$\Downarrow$
Active force per mm^2	$\Downarrow$	$\Downarrow$ or =
Energetics		

Curvature G of F/V curve	⇑	⇑
Contractile and membrane proteins		
Action potential duration	⇑	⇑
Ca transient duration	⇑	⇑
Isomyosin shift to V3	+	+
Ca^{2+} ATPase of SR	⇓	⇓
Na^+/Ca^{2+} exchanger	⇑	?
$\alpha 3\ Na^+, K^+$ ATPase	+	+

Note: * Significant differences between senescence and overload. ⇓ decreased, ⇑ enhanced, = unchanged, + pronounced, +++ extremely important, ? controversial.

Biological determinants of myocardial function at rest

Systolic function

The Baltimore study has clearly demonstrated that cardiac output, at rest, is unaltered with age. Aortic impedance is greatly increased with aging mainly because of an increased aortic stiffness and diameter [Tedgui et Levy 1994]. During senescence the enhanced characteristic impedance of the aorta is responsible for a left ventricular overload, which in turn activates the expression of several specific genes, as detailed below.

Action potential and the myoplasmic calcium transient are also prolonged. Studies of the contractility of papillary muscle were complicated by the fact that the senescent papillary muscle is both thicker and stiffer than the young muscles. Nevertheless, it has been shown that isometric as well as isotonic contraction is prolonged in every species studied and that both the maximum velocity of shortening and the maximum unloaded shortening velocity are depressed (Table 3. 4). Relaxation is also impaired.

Table 3. 5. Senescent heart versus overloaded heart: ANS, RAS, and ANF

	Overloaded	Senescence
Autonomous nervous system		
β-adrenergic receptors	⇓	= or ⇓
mRNA	⇓	⇓⇓
Muscarinic receptors	⇓	⇓⇓*
mRNA	⇓	⇑
$G_{\alpha s}$	=	⇓
$G_{\alpha i}$	=	=
Adenylate cyclase activity	⇓	⇓
Renin-angiotensin system		
Circulating	⇑	⇓⇓*
Myocardial	⇑	*
Atrial natriuretic factor		
Plasma levels	⇑	⇑
LV mRNA	⇑	⇑

* Significant differences between senescence and overload. Note: ⇓ decreased, ⇑ enhanced, = unchanged.

Active force per surface area is correlated with the biochemical parameters and more particularly with the isomyosin shift which suggests that this parameter reflects, in part, the state of contractility. All these modifications were similar to those observed during pressure overload. Moreover, the skinned myofilament response to calcium was unaltered, suggesting that the changes in the velocity of contraction that have been observed depend on contractile proteins and/or the intracellular calcium movements. The slowing of the contraction allows the senescent muscle to maintain the active tension within the normal limits but to the detriment of the velocity at which this tension is developed. Both physiological and biochemical changes have therefore a beneficial effect in terms of muscle energetics. Contraction energetics of the papillary muscle were calculated from mechanical parameters that had indicated that each contraction was more economical [Besse et al. 1993]. An interesting finding, made in humans [Hasenfuss et al. 1992], is the fact that the force-time integral of the individual myosin cross-bridge cycle correlates with the age of patients with nonfailing myocardium, suggesting that, even in humans, aging is associated with an improvement of contraction economy.

In the rat ventricle, the isomyosin content shifts progressively with age from V1 to V3. The modifications of the membrane proteins occur at several different levels, including the Ca^{2+} ATPase of SR, adrenergic and vagal receptors, calcium channels, the Na^+/Ca^{2+} exchange [Heyliger et al. 1988] and the Na^+, K^+-ATPase (unpublished data from our laboratory). This phenoconversion of the membrane proteins is directly responsible for the slowing of the intracellular calcium transient [Orchard and Lakatta 1985] and is very similar to what has been reported to occur during mechanical overload (Figure 3. 2).

Diastolic function

During senescence the global diastolic function remains unchanged in spite of a pronounced impairment in the early ventricular filling because the contribution of atrial systole to ventricular filling is increased [Fleg 1987; Lakatta 1993]. The impairment in early ventricular filling and the diminution of the E wave shown by EchoDoppler results from both a prolonged active isovolumic relaxation and an increased myocardial stiffness. Thus, a 50% reduction in the rate of left ventricular filling during early diastole is observed between 30 to 80 years. Active relaxation is altered by senescence. As explained above, myocardial fibrosis is an important component of the senescent heart and is responsible for the major changes in passive compliance in both heart and vessels. The origin of fibrosis in the senescent heart is debatable, and the most likely hypothesis is that it is replacement fibrosis due to myocyte loss [Eghbali et al. 1980; Besse et al. 1993]. During senescence atrial hypertrophy and a slowing of atrial contraction compensates for the impairment in the early diastolic filling.

The cardiovascular response to exercise

In elderly people, during exercise the maximal cardiac output is maintained by an increased ejection fraction and an increased utilization of the Frank-Starling mechanism with only slight tachycardia, or no increase in the heart rate at all. There also is evidence that the responsiveness to catecholamines is attenuated.

In the senescent rat heart, the density of both the total number of β-adrenergic and muscarinic receptors is reduced; however, the decrease in muscarinic receptor density is greater than that in total β-adrenergic receptors [Chevalier et al. 1991; Hardouin et al. 1993]. A similar decrease in the number of muscarinic receptors has also been reported in the cerebral cortex, striatum, and hippocampus, suggesting that, for unknown reasons, aging has a rather specific and pronounced effect on the muscarinic system [Danner and Halbrook 1990]. Aging, as mechanical overload, is accompanied by several modifications of the ANS that are likely to be located "down the road," as initially suggested by E. Lakatta [1993] (Table 3. 5).

Arrhythmias

Clinical and experimental studies that have examined cardiac rhythm in a healthy geriatric population, carefully evaluated to exclude cardiac disease, demonstrate a prevalence of supraventricular and ventricular ectopic beats [Fleg and Kennedy 1982]. Time domain analysis has also shown that the standard deviation of the R-R interval decreases with age [Schwartz et al. 1991].

In the senescent heart, arrhythmias result from both fibrosis and changes in the membrane phenotype. Fibrosis is undoubtedly a major factor of reentry and also auriculoventricular block. Moreover, it may create centers of automaticity. The intracellular calcium transient peaks normally but is prolonged, and the duration of the action potential is increased. These two factors are potentially arrhythmogenic. Studies on the L-type calcium current are still rare in senescent myocytes. Only a small increase in the peak current density associated with a reduced inactivation has been demonstrated.

Cardiac hormones

Plasma ANF levels are elevated in healthy elderly people as compared with young individuals, but the factors responsible for these differences are still poorly known. Old rats also have higher plasma ANF levels (Table 3. 5) than young rats. In vitro the basal ANF secretory rate and the secretory response to phenylephrine (but not the response to stretch) were greater in atria from aged animals, suggesting that an increased secretory response to adrenergic stimulation may contribute to the enhanced ANF plasma levels. Molecular biological determination of the relative levels of mRNA coding for ANF showed a strong activation in the left but not in the right ventricle [Heymes et al. 1994].

Aging in humans, and rat (Table 3.5) is associated with low plasma levels of angio I, renin activity, and angiotensinogen. The latter is likely to reflect a diminution in the hepatic level of angiotensinogen mRNA. In contrast, the myocardial mRNA levels for both angiotensinogen and angiotensin converting enzyme were both upregulated. This upregulation is restricted to the left ventricle and does not exist in the right ventricle [Corman and Michel 1986; Heymes et al. 1994].

Both angiotensinogen and its mRNA are rather abundant in the atria but nearly absent in the ventricles of young animals. In young rats ACE is present and active but rather poorly expressed. During mechanical overload, plasma ANF increases, and the ANF mRNA is activated in the overloaded ventricle. The myocardial renin-angiotensin-system, including angiotensinogen and the angiotensin receptors, is also activated after a prolonged mechanical stress. During senescence, the specific left ventricular activation of normally poorly expressed genes - such as the genes coding for ANF, angiotensinogene, and ACE - suggests that the trigger for activation is common to the two systems and is in fact a left ventricular mechanical overload.

Senescence is known to be associated with several other changes in the hormonal status: (1) the plasma level in free T4 was depressed, but that of T3, which is the active thyroid hormone, was not; (2) the plasma cortisol levels were increased, but aldosterone remained unchanged in spite of a pronounced down-regulation of the RAS. Both findings have been fully documented in humans.

CF is mainly a disease of the elderly, and the average age of the patients of most of the clinical trials, including the CONSENSUS study on angiotensin converting enzyme inhibitor (CEI) is around 65 years. Obviously, most of the patients under CEI have a very low level of plasma angio I, and there is a question about how CEI works in the elderly. The answer is most likely to be found in the various tissue renin-angiotensin-systems, at least the one located in the myocardium, as already suggested [Heymes et al. 1995, Heymes et al. 1998].

Protein synthesis

During aging the rate of both protein synthesis and degradation decrease in parallel in the heart as in others tissues, but the myocardial total RNA content remains unchanged [Danner and Holbrook 1990). The recent availability of molecular biology techniques allows the quantitation of both the concentration of total polyA containing RNA (i.e. mRNAs) and specific mRNA. Data from this laboratory have shown that both the yield of total RNA and the total amount of cardiac mRNAs (or polyA containing RNAs) relative to ribosomal RNA remain unchanged.

The main problem, in the heart as in other tissues, is the relative quantification of a given mRNA. Cardiac senescence is accompanied by several changes in genetic expression: (1) There are shifts in the expression of isogenes, such as those coding for α and β myosin heavy chains (α-myosin heavy chain mRNA disappears and is replaced by the isomRNA β). (2) The relative concentration (in mg per mg) in other mRNAs, such as that encoding the Ca^{2+} ATPase of the SR decreases, suggesting that these genes are rather inactive during senescence and that, consequently, the corresponding protein and mRNA are diluted in a heart whose mass is increased. The total cardiac content (in g per heart), in protein (or mRNA) belonging to this family of genes remains unchanged. (3) Nevertheless there are also genes such as collagen and the β1-adrenergic receptor (Table 3. 5) whose expression is likely to be decreased during senescence. In this family both the concentration and the total amount of mRNA per heart are decreased, but there is additional evidence of a post-transcriptional regulation. (4) Finally, as explained below, there are, in the myocardium and very likely in the cardiac myocytes, at least 3 genes that are activated during senescence - namely the genes encoding the ANF, Angen, and ACE.

The modifications in both protein synthesis and degradation [Crie et al. 1981] and mRNA content that occur during aging would suggest that the senescent heart may also be unable to adapt to an increased load and would be unable to further hypertrophy in response to a mechanical stress. This question is of more than an academic interest since both arterial hypertension and coronary insufficiency, the two main causes of cardiac hypertrophy and failure, are indeed much more frequent after 65 years than before. Several experimental investigators have tried to answer this question [Capasso et al. 1986; Isoyama et al. 1987]. Although the results were somewhat contradictory, the general opinion is that the senescent heart responds more slowly to mechanical overload than the young hearts but that the final result is the same in terms of myocardial mass [Besse et al. 1993].

The genetics of aging

While genetics of aging is not a specific problem for cardiovascular research, it is important to know about the recent progress made in this domain to better understand what we are observing into the myocardium. The heritability of lifespan is small in human and in animals: for example, twins who have been reared separately do not share an heritable lifespan [Finch and Tanzi 1997]. Experimental manipulations of lifespan showed that several genes may have positive or negative impacts on the duration of life, including *wg* in fruifly antennae, longevity-determining genes in yeast, *age-1* which doubles life-span in nematodes, the E2 allele of Apolipoprotein E (see below), the gene responsible for the Werner syndrome (which is like a DNA helicase and genes involved in age-related neurodegenerative disorders like the Alzheimer's disease). Nevertheless, the genetic determination of lifespan cannot be equated with the action of an even complicated genetic programme, and the role of genetic factors remains minor as compared to environmental parameters, including oxidative stress and caloric restriction. The latter point, which may obviously interest the clinician, is that for the moment the best way to increase lifespan in mice is caloric restriction [Sohal and Weindruch 1997] - an awful perspective, for a frenchman !

The senescent heart, a diseased heart

As explained previously, careful and detailed clinical investigations have demonstrated that the senescent heart has normal myocardial performances at rest and during exercising because it uses several compensatory mechanisms to maintain a normal output [Assayag et al. 1997b]. Experimental investigations have shown several modifications both at the cellular and molecular levels in the aging rat heart, which are very similar to those observed during experimental pressure overload including a slowing of the action potential, the calcium transient and contraction associated with an isomyosin shift to the V3 isoform, a diminished density or activity of the calcium ATPase of SR and Na^+/Ca^{2+} exchange, and a reduced activity of the adrenergic system.

Fibrosis is also a common feature found during both overload and in senescence. Nevertheless, although fibrosis is a constant finding in the aged heart, there are several clinical and experimental examples of mechanically overloaded hearts in which the collagen concentration remains normal. It has recently been suggested that fibrosis in these particular conditions is under hormonal control. Arrhythmias and a loss in heart rate variability are a common feature found in both conditions in human and in animals. Nevertheless, the types of arrhythmias, their frequency, and their prognostic value are extremely different.

The β-adrenergic/muscarinic receptor ratio remains unchanged during compensated cardiac hypertrophy, while the same ratio is reduced during senescence in the rat heart due to a much more pronounced decrease in muscarinic compared to β-adrenergic receptor density. Molecular biological data suggest that the mode of regulation is different.

4

GENETICS FOR NON GENETICIANS

DNA POLYMORPHISM

Definitions

Slight variations in the DNA occur in approximately one of every 3,000 bp. In humans, this roughly represents 1 million differences between two unrelated individuals. DNA polymorphism determines genotypic polymorphism, which may be translated into phenotypic polymorphism (Figure 1. 1), but not necessarily so. DNA polymorphism may indeed be silent and will not cause any phenotypic change. Such changes would either occur in an irrelevant part of the gene or would not change the properties of the encoding protein (remember, for example, that several triplets may code for the same aminoacid). Such a polymorphism is widely used for linkage analysis and polymorphic sites are used as markers. Conventionally, polymorphism is restricted to allelic variations occurring with a frequency >1%; rare variants or mutations qualify allelic variations occurring at a frequency of <1%. Polymorphism can also occur within the gene, either in the coding part of the gene or in the regulatory part upstream of the first exon, and is the cause of a genetic disease, if the mutation gives rise to a defective protein or even inhibits gene expression. Nevertheless, and fortunately for us, DNA polymorphism rarely gives rise to a disease because most of the mutations do not result in a phenotypic change.

DNA polymorphism can be punctual and then is identifiable after DNA sequencing, which is a rather long job. Punctual polymorphism can be located on a restriction site. It then modifies a restriction site and the corresponding restriction map (Figure 1. 14) and generates restriction fragments of different lengths: it is termed restriction fragment length polymorphism (RFLP).

Allele has usually been used to qualify DNA polymorphism in the coding part of a gene.The word is now more widely used to qualify polymorphism located either in a gene or in the anonymous part of the genome. As illustrated in figure 4. 1. during cell division there are 2 copies of allele 1, one on each chromatid of the same father's chromosome, there are also 2 copies of allele 2 on the mother's chromosome. A diseased gene is also the allelic variant of a normal gene. Variants located at a restriction site reflect restriction polymorphism (Figure 4. 2.). Alleles can be closed one to each other as allele 1/2 and allele 3/4 on figure 4. 2. They are termed *haplotype*, and then the alleles cosegregate. Haplotypes are not randomly inherited: they are linked, and the linkage is therefore in disequilibrium.

Repetitive polymorphism is different. It has no physiological consequences but represents a major tool for exploring the genome. There are indeed individual differences in repeated di- and trinucleotides termed short tandem repeats (STR) or microsatellites. This polymorphism is easily detectable by PCR (see figure 4. 7) by using two primers flanking the repeated units to sequentially amplify the STR. The resulting amplification products have different sizes and can be separated by gel electrophoresis. Figure 4. 7. shows two alleles - one with 4 repeats on the father's chromosome and the other with 6 repeats on the mother's chromosome. This difference in size can be used to track the inheritance of each chromosome and the degree of linkage of these alleles with a diseased gene.

215

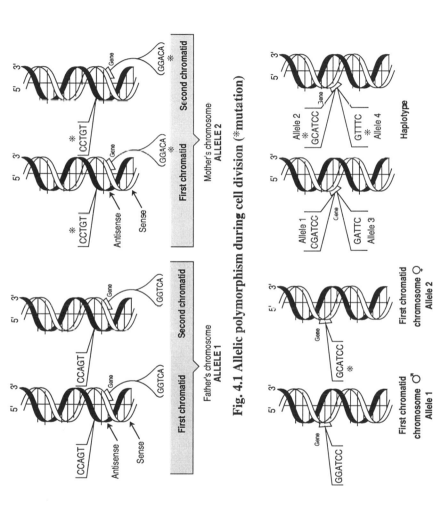

Fig. 4.1 Allelic polymorphism during cell division (*mutation)

Fig. 4.2. Restriction polymorphism on Bam H1 (left) and haplotype (Allele 1 + 3 or 2 + 4) (right)

What causes DNA polymorphism?

Tchernobyl had certainly caused mutations, and, presently, the impredicitible evolution of humanity can unfortunately allow us to predict that genetics has chances to become a major health problem. Nevertheless, for the moment, most mutations do not result from physical or chemical injuries but are consequences of the normal mixing of the genetic material during meiosis and more specifically during the crossing-over (Figure 4. 3). The genetic consequences of meiosis in terms of mixing genetic material are the following: (1) after the first meiotic division the homologous chromosomes segregate into the daughter cells randomly with regard to parental origin; (2) during middle prophase I homologous chromosomes synapse and crossing-over between chromatids of homologous chromosomes occurs, but synapses do not necessarily coincide (Figure 4. 3); (3) chromatids assort randomly into the daughter cells; (4) in mammals, in the male, each of the 4 haploid cells produced by meiosis give rise to a sperm cell, whereas in the female only one of the haploid cells survives as an egg nucleus; the fusion of an egg and a sperm gives rise to a new diploid cell.

Any two genes, or *loci*, that are on the same chromosome are also by definition on the same DNA molecule. They are both therefore, to a certain extent, linked. Nevertheless, as illustrated on Figure 4. 4, if two loci (the locus of a polymorphic marker - namely, a tandem repeat - and that of the diseased gene) are located far apart on the chromosome, recombination events have more chances to occur than if they are close together.

The genetic distance is the distance that separates the two loci from each other. It is expressed in *cMorgans* (cM). cMs are statistical units: 1 cM is equal to 1% recombination during crossing-over. The likelihood of having a crossing-over that separates 2 loci whose genetic distance is 1cM is therefore one chance in a 100. Strictly speaking, genetic distance is not a physical unit; nevertheless 1 cM roughly corresponds to 1 million bp. In

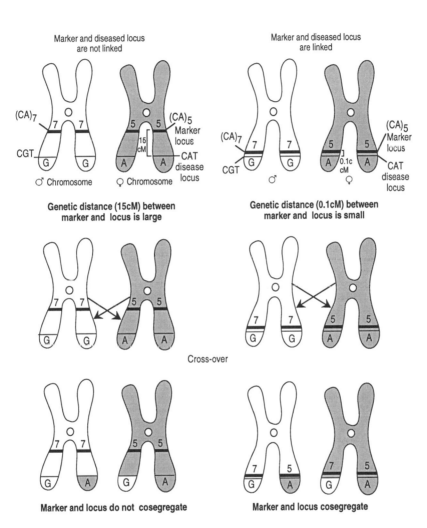

Fig. 4.3. The physical basis of genetic linkage during meiosis

218

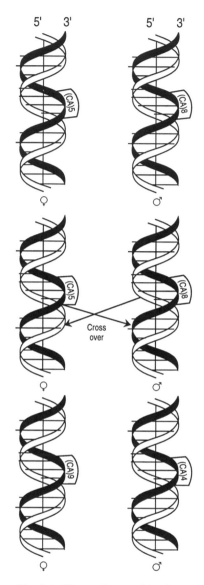

Fig. 4.4.   Unequal recombination

Figure 4. 4, the 2 loci that are 15 cM apart are poorly linked, and the marker provides very little information concerning the place where the diseased locus is located. The marker is then said to be poorly informative. In contrast, if the distance is 0.1 cM, which means that the marker is close to the diseased gene (it may, for example, be located in the intron of the diseased gene as in Cambien et al. 1992), it would be an informative marker.

Figure 4. 4 shows one example of how a genetic variant of tandem repeats can be created. During synapsis, the hybridation of the tandem repeats is slightly shifted downward, and the resulting new chromosomes obtained after the crossing-over have different repeats: $(CA)_9$ for the father's chromosome instead of $(CA)_5$, and $(CA)_4$ for the mother's instead of $(CA)_8$. Genetic conversion is another example of recombination that results from the triggering of the reparative process (Figure 4. 5). Random assignment of alleles after crossing-over may result in *mismatches*, or *mispairing*, which means that a given pair of bases will no longer be complementary on the DNA strands. Spontaneously, a reparative process starts within the nucleus, which uses the complementary strand as a guide but the process is random and may use, as a guide, either DNA strand. The result is a rather complex mixture of new variants.

What are the consequences of DNA polymorphism?

DNA polymorphism may create genetic diseases but is mainly beneficial in terms of evolution, since it produces diversity. Several of the processes above-described that create polymorphism are also mechanisms responsible for biological regulations such as alternative splicing, which is also used to modulate the expression of isoforms, or unequal recombinations which is likely to be at the origin of several of the superfamilies of membrane proteins (Figure 4. 4. and Table 1. 9).

220

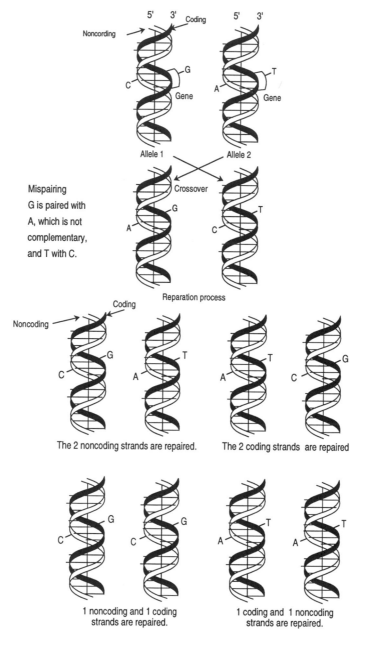

Fig. 4.5. Genetic conversion

INHERITED DISEASES

Strategies to isolate a mutation

Classical genetics

Classical genetics starts from a candidate protein which is supposed to be the probable diseased protein. Familial anemia, for example, was thought to be due to mutations within hemoglobin. The gene encoding the hemoglobin subunits was cloned and the mutation responsible for sickle cell anemia was discovered. Unfortunately, in most cases the working hypothesis is too vague or broad and other approaches like positional cloning, frequently termed *reverse genetics*, and populational approach are necessary (Figure 4. 6).

Reverse genetics

Reverse genetics is based solely on the knowledge that the disease is monogenic and heritable and that there is a familial approach. Search for the genetic location of the disease consists in testing many randomly chosen DNA markers until one is found that segregates with the disease, which means that the 2 DNA segments, the marker and the diseased gene, are linked - that is physically located close to each other on the same chromosome arm. The challenge then is to detect a mutation, which is a unique base substitution, in the genome that consists of roughly 100,000 genes and is approximately 3 billion bp long (Table 1. 2), and then to localize the mutation within a chromosome that is, on average, 120 million bp long. Finding the mutation can be compared to looking for a needle in a huge haystack! Such a scale explains, for example, why the final identification of the mutation responsible for cystic fibrosis was so long and needed so many people and so much funding and effort.

Reverse genetics consists in evaluating the genetic distance that separates the diseased gene from informative markers (Figure 4. 1). There are, for the moment, certainly more than a thousand markers of known chromosomal location, and the number is increasing day by day. In addition, the mapping of the human genome is progressing rapidly.

Markers are important, but the availability of well-characterized families with numerous affected members is also determinant. In addition, a major issue, especially in cardiovascular research, is the relevance of clinical data. The clinical phenotype has to be extremely well-defined *a priori*, and not *a posteriori*: criteria for a normal blood pressure, a myocardial infarction, and exclusion criteria need to be rigorously defined long before starting the genetic study.

Statistical analysis is then utilized to establish whether a given marker is linked to the disease or if the linkage is only occasional. The recombination frequency, q, between two loci is equal to the percentage of recombinants obtained divided by the total number of meiosis that have been examined and is expressed in cM. $q = 0$ means that the marker and the diseased locus are closely linked and may be identical. $q = 0.50$ means that the 2 loci are not linked and can only cosegregate randomly, i.e. in 50% of the cases according to the Mendel's laws. They are located on different chromosomes, the genetic distance is above 50 cM, and linkage is unlikely. The statistical analysis consists in calculating the likelihood that the 2 loci are linked at given recombination frequencies q = 0.1, 0.3, 0.4, 0.5. The result is expressed in log as LOD score Z, and a curve is drawn by plotting q as a function of Z. The recombination fraction giving the highest LOD score is thus the relation with the highest probability to be the true value. By convention, a LOD score >3 is considered as significant and a LOD score >3 for $q = 0.13$ means that the hypothesis that the 2 loci are linked at a genetical distance of $q = 13$ cM is 10^3 (1,000 times) times more likely

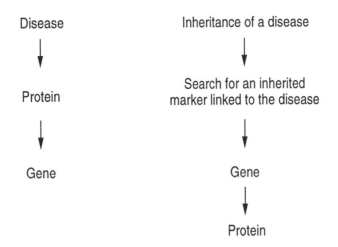

Fig. 4.6. **Strategies for identifying diseased genes**

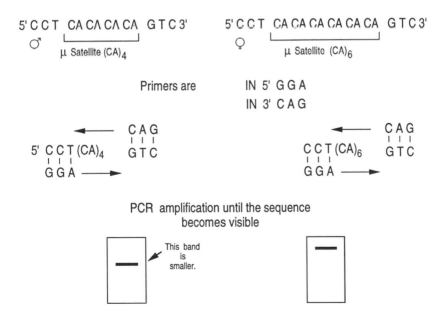

Fig. 4.7. **Short tandem repeats identification by PCR (repetition polymorphism or micro satellites)**

that the opposite hypothesis. In contrast, the LOD score analysis also allows one to exclude a linkage if the LOD score < - 2 .

The next step is to ascertain the physical distance between the diseased locus and the different markers and finally to isolate and clone the gene and the mutation. The latter may require years of work and needs precise strategy which is beyond the scope of this book Interestingly there are numerous examples of genetic diseases that have resulted in the discovery of new genes and new proteins. Two good examples are cystic fibrosis, which allowed the discovery of a chloride channel, and the Duchenne muscular dystrophy, which is due to mutations in dystrophin (Figure 2. 15) (Kaplan et Delpech 1993).

Populational approach (candidate gene)

In multifactorial diseases, the phenotype results from the expression of multiple genes, which renders segregation studies as described above difficult to interpret. In the populational approach, it is mandatory to have a good candidate gene. DNA markers located on the responsible gene itself or within close proximity are then used, and the frequency of the marker in the diseased population is then compared to that of a control population (Soubrier and Cambien 1993). Several candidate genes have already been selected for such a purpose, as angiotensinogen or ACE to study arterial hypertension, or as apolipoproteins to study hyperlipidemia.

Positional candidate strategy

As more sequences have been identified and entered into databases (see above), it will make it easier to assign such candidate gene. Hence, the 2 above-described methods will converge to what is called a *positional candidate approch* [Collins 1995]. Such a method uses database screening as a tool to explore the diseased part of the chromosome, which has been

225

previously identified by positional cloning. The culprit gene can be subsequently examined by PCR.

Main types of hereditary diseases

Hereditary diseases are diseases due to a mutation occurring on one or several genes. Figure 4. 8 summarizes the main categories of genetic diseases.

(1) Monogenic diseases with a founder effect are due to a single mutation that results in the absence of one amino acid and both a defective protein and function. The mutation may be historically unique. The most well-known example is sickle cell anemia, which is due to a mutation in codon 6 of the β-globin gene. This mutation results in the substitution of a negative amino acid, glutamic acid, by a neutral residue, valine. Individuals bearing such a mutation also possess the same genetic markers of the locus which allows one to say that the accident occurred only once in one founder. The mutation creates a disease, anemia, but it also protects these people against malaria, which explains why such a unique event has finally been disseminated throughout Africa.

Mutation is dominant when the clinical manifestations are seen in heterozygotous patients and recessive when clinical signs need to be expressed homozygous (Figure 4. 9). Autosomal means that the disease gene is carried by any of the 22 chromosomes that are not chromosome X or Y. When mutations are linked to chromosome X, clinical manifestations are linked to sex and present only in boys. Nevertheless, girls carry the mutation and will transmit the disease to their male progeny.

There are also monogenic monoallelic diseases with a founder effect that are due to the same mutation. Nevertheless, because the mutation is not always linked to the same markers, it is possible to conclude that the disease originated from several identical accidents occurring in different places at

226

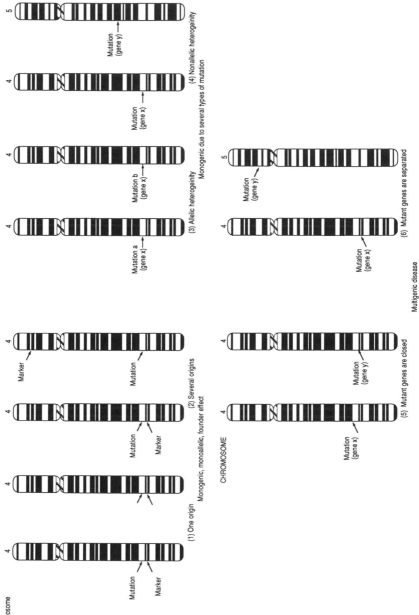

Fig. 4.8. Monogenic and multigenic hereditary diseases

different moments (Figure 4. 8). In these conditions both phenotype and genotype are unique.

(2) Most of the monogenic diseases are, however, due to several different mutations. The phenotype is identical, but the genotypes are different. It is possible to have different mutations on the same gene, resulting in the same clinical syndrome. This situation is termed *allelic heterogeineity*. Familial hypercholesterolemia, for example, may result from approximately 200 different mutations on the lipoprotein receptor gene. There are also nonallelic heterogeineity - that is mutations occurring on different genes, on different chromosomes (Figure 4. 8), but again giving rise to the same phenotype. A good example is familial hypertrophic cardiomyopathy which may be due to mutations on, at the least, five different chromosomes.

(3) Multigenic diseases are due to several mutations that can be genetically linked or, by contrast, located on different chromosomes. Arterial hypertension, hyperlipidemias, and diabetes belong to this category. Atherosclerosis is determined by the combination of the above diseases, plus additional genetic factors, plus environmental factors. Atherosclerosis is then both multigenic and multifactorial. Such extreme complexity has suggested an entirely different strategy to geneticians who want to begin research in the cardiovascular field.

To reduce the problem to manageable dimensions, genetic studies have focused on the study of intermediate *traits* that were previously identified as risk factors in terms of clinical manifestations of atherosclerosis as coronary artery disease (CAD). Nevertheless such traits, such as arterial hypertension, diseases of hemostasis, hyperlipidemias or diabetes, are still extremely complex. There are, for example, at least 200 genes that are involved in lipid metabolism and in which mutations may be responsible for hyperlipidemias. The "genetic architecture" [Sing and Moll 1990] responsible for the distribution of a trait in a large population is defined by the number of genes and alleles responsible for the expression of that trait, but it also includes the impact of alleles on the level of the trait and its relationship with other risk factors. The effort spent on trying to present a complete genetic architecture of inherited risk factors is great, especially in hyperlipidemias, but for the moment an overall picture is still lacking even for one identifiable trait.

Genotype and phenotype relationships

When someone is not fully involved in genetics, it is quite common to think that a given mutation will automatically result in a given specific phenotype and that exceptions to this rule are exceptional. This is completely wrong [Benlian 1996]. One of the best examples is familial hypercholesterolemia due to a deficit in the clearance of the low density lipoproteins (LDLs). The clinical manifestations of the disease are nearly indistinguishable whether the disease is caused by mutations at the LDL receptor level (and there are approximately 200 of them) or at the level of the apoprotein B-100 - that is the substrate itself. The same is true for familial hypertrophic cardiomyopathies. The same clinical signs are observed whether the mutation is on myosin or on thin filament proteins. Good examples are also detectable in familial obesity and familial arterial hypertension.

Strictly speaking, the opposite is not true, and the same mutation cannot generate different phenotypes. Nevertheless there are number of examples of inherited diseases in which different clinical manifestations may originate from mutations on the same gene, on the same locus. For example, mutations at the level of the apoprotein A-1 may result in hypoglyceridemia, hyperglyceridemia, amylosis, neuropathy and so on.

229

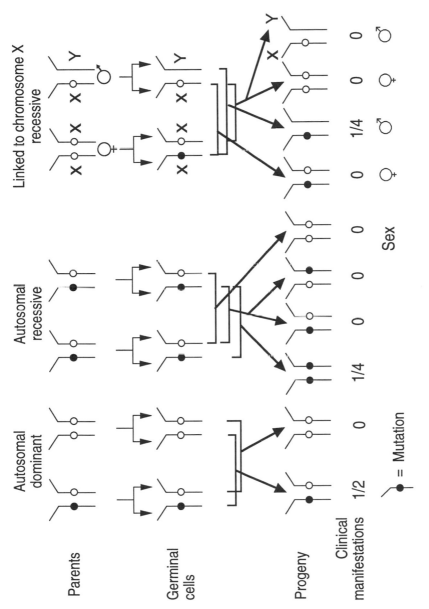

Fig. 4.9. Modes of inheritance

Inherited cardiovascular diseases and risk factors

Cardiology has been for a long time more closely linked to environmental problems than to genetics. Sudden death was more often attributed to diet or smoking than to heredity. Genetic epidemiology is a rather new branch of cardiology and data comparing heritability to environmental factors are still rare, although concordant. At present, although it is possible to provide sufficient data to convince cardiologists that genetics will soon become a major tool for preventing, diagnosing and perhaps treating cardiovascular diseases, it is impossible to write an extensive review of the subject.

The goal of this chapter is therefore to illustrate the new ways that have been recently suggested by a few pioneer publications. For the moment, an extensive review of genetics in cardiology is likely to be an impossible task. The reader interested inhaving more complete information in this field should read the following reviews (Breslow 1993; Chan et al. 1990; Sing and Moll 1990; Soubrier and Cambien 1993; Corvol and Charru 1993).

There are, as yet, several cardiovascular diseases that are monogenic, such as familial cardiomyopathy (FCM) and there is only one that is both monogenic and monoallelic, the familial defective apo B-100. The strategy that has been used to explore the genetic factors in cardiovascular diseases is different from that commonly applied to problems such as cystic fibrosis or hemoglobinopathies. For similar reasons, this approach is also used for cancer and asthma. In this chapter, an attempt has been made to start with rather simple problems, those arising from monogenic diseases, and then to establish a few bases for the study of more complex problems.

231

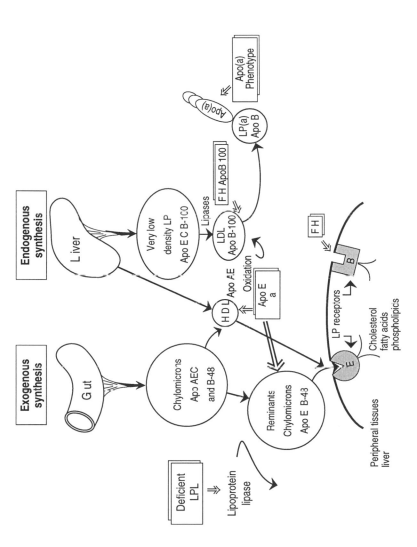

Fig. 4.10. Pathways for lipid transport and main mechanisms for hyperlipidemias (in boxes)
LP : lipoproteins. Receptors E and B : receptors for Apo E and B of corresponding LPs

MONOGENIC CARDIOVASCULAR DISEASES

Familial defective apo B-100, FDA

FDA is a frequent (1: 500) autosomal dominant monogenic and, for the moment, the only monoallelic (as drepanocytose) familial cardiovascular disease what has been unambiguously identified. Whether the mutation originates from one or several places in the world is unknown. Hyperlipidemia is caused by an increased level of LDL cholesterol level and is associated with premature atherosclerosis. Such a type of hyperlipidemia is due to a defective clearance in LDL, and familial defective apo B-100 is one of the forms of type IIa hyperlipidemia.

The is caused by a mutation in the coding sequence of the apo-B gene (on chromosome 2, 2p24) that changes an arginine codon at amino acid 3,500 to glutamine [Tybjaerg-Hansen and Humphries 1992]. The apo-B gene (14 kb) is unique and composed of 27 very small exons (around 175 kb) + exon 26 and exon 29, that are 2 enormous exons located at the 3' end of the gene (7,572 and 1,906 kb). This unique gene express 2 different isoforms by RNA editing, apo B-100 (as 100%) which is synthetized in the liver and apo B-48 (48% smaller) which is produced into the intestin and forms the proteic part of chylomicrons (Figure 4. 10). A specific cytidine deaminase is indeed able to create a codon-stop on position 6,666, which interrupts the maturation process and alllows the production of these 2 isoforms with different lengths.

The LDL receptor-binding region of apo-B is located in 3' and is not expressed in apo B-48. The mutated codon is also located in 3', on apo B-100, and the mutation results in a protein with a very low affinity for the receptor. LDL are lipoproteins that contain apo-B100 after lipolysis of very low density lipoproteins. LDL deliver cholesterol to the liver and peripheral tissues (Figure 4. 10). Their cellular uptake is mediated by the LDL receptors that recognize apo-B100. The disease is monoallelic and therefore easily detectable by routine analysis on spotted whole blood using PCR amplification [Hansen et al. 1991]. The technique used by Peter Hansen is an interesting clinical application of PCR and consists of introducing a cleavage site for the restriction enzyme MspI (C/CGG) in normal alleles but not in mutant alleles (Fig. 4. 11).

Familial hypercholesterolemia

This disease is frequent (1: 500 for heterozygotes) autosomal dominant monogenic, but multiallelic and should be better called *defective lipoprotein receptor familial hypercholesterolemia*, since, as explained above, the phenotype is the same as described previously for FDA - that is hypercholesterolemia with premature atherosclerosis - and is associated with the occurrence of planar xantoma in the homozygous forms. This is also a type IIa hyperlipidemia with a defective clearance of LDL, nevertheless in this case the structure of apoliproteine B is unchanged and the mutation is located on the LDL receptors. The human LDL receptor gene is unique on chromosome 19p13.2, spans 45 kb and has 18 exons (Figure 4. 12).

The first mutations were reported by two Noble prize winners [Brown and Goldstein 1986]. Nearly 200 different mutations have now been reported. The mutations are located all along the gene and can result in the total absence of receptor (class 1) or a deficiency in the transport of the newly synthetized receptor (class 2), in the lipoprotein fixation (class 3), in the process of receptor internalization (class 4), or in the recycling process (class 5). Such a multiallelism renders the routine detection of the diseased mutation tedious and necessitates the alternate approach of linkage analysis.

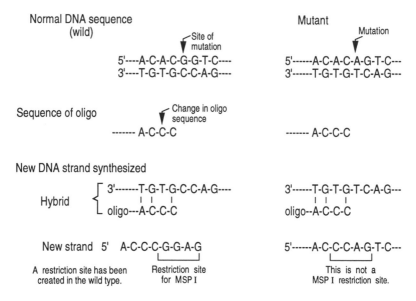

Normal DNA sequence
(wild)

Site of mutation

5'----A-C-A-C-G-G-T-C----
3'----T-G-T-G-C-C-A-G----

Mutant

Mutation

5'------A-C-A-C-A-G-T-C---
3'------T-G-T-G-T-C-A-G---

Sequence of oligo

Change in oligo sequence

------- A-C-C-C

------- A-C-C-C

New DNA strand synthesized

Hybrid { 3'-------T-G-T-G-C-C-A-G----
           | | |
        oligo---A-C-C-C

3'------T-G-T-G-T-C-A-G---
         | | |
oligo--A-C-C-C

New strand 5' A-C-C-C-G-G-A-G

A restriction site has been created in the wild type.

Restriction site for MSP I

5'------A-C-C-C-A-G-T-C---

This is not a MSP I restriction site.

Fig. 4.11. Detection of the apo B - 3,500 mutation by PCR on blood spots

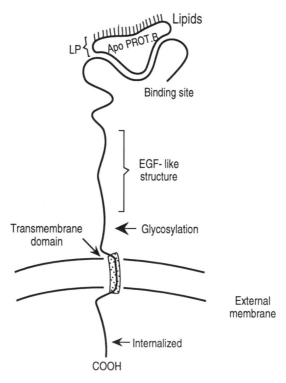

Lipids

LP { Apo PROT.B

Binding site

EGF- like structure

Transmembrane domain

← Glycosylation

External membrane

← Internalized

COOH

Fig. 4.12. Lipoprotein (LP) receptor [from Brown and Goldstein 1986]

Mendelian forms of arterial hypertension

Glucocorticoid-remediable aldosteronism is an autosomal dominant trait charcterized by hypertension and a hyperaldosteronism [Lifton 1996]. The disease is caused by a novel gene that results from duplications arising from unequal crossing-over between the aldosynthase and 11β-hydroxylase genes, fusing 5' regulatory sequences from the latter onto coding sequences from the other. By virtue of this fusion the aldosynthase is brought under the control of ACTH, which results in ectopic secretion of aldosterone from the adrenal fasciculata. Aldosterone secretion then becomes insensitive to plasma volume. Carriers can be treated by glucocorticoids, which suppress ACTH secretion.

The syndrome of apparent mineralocorticoid excess is an autosomal recessive form of hypertension with low levels of aldosterone. It may be caused by mutations on the 11 β-hydroxysteroid dehydrogenase - the enzyme that is linked to mineralocorticoid receptors and protects the receptors from cortisol by metabolizing cortisol to cortisone.

The Liddle's syndrome is an inherited form of hypertension that is caused by gain-of-function mutations. Mutations are indeed localized on genes encoding the subunits of the amiloride-sensitive kidney ENaC channel. They result in an increased sodium reabsorption and explain the hypertension seen in the patients who carry the mutation.

Familial cardiomyopathies

The definition of *cardiomyopathy* in contemporary use remains one of exclusion cardiomyopathies are heart muscle diseases of unknown cause, cardiopathy usually qualifies cardiac disease of known origin as ischemic or hypertensive cardiopathy. In fact, advances in biology have modified the definition, and cardiomyopathies are now defined as diseases of the heart in the absence of coronary disease, hypertension, congenital anatomic distortion, or valve disease. The definition therefore includes cardiomyopathies of unknown causes; cardiomyopathies due to infections, toxins, poisons, drugs, and metabolic disorders; and inherited cardiomyopathies.

Familial hypertrophic cardiomyopathies (FHC)

Hypertrophic cardiomyopathy is familial in half of the cases and sporadic in the other half. FHC usually has an autosomal dominant pattern of inheritance (a few cases of autosomal recessive or nonautosomal, X-linked and recessive patterns of inheritance have been reported). The incidence of the disease is around 2.5 per 100,000 inhabitants per year. The penetrance of FHC is incomplete in young individuals and increases with age. The disease is severe, and the annual mortality rate is 2 to 4%.

FHC is characterized by a primary myocardial hypertrophy that is most frequently asymmetric. Two major specific features characterize the disease: (1) a high incidence of ventricular tachycardia and sudden death (the disease is one of the major causes of sudden death in athletes); (2) a normal systolic function with an accelerated ejection velocity and pronounced diastolic dysfunction. Histological examination reveals an increased myocardial mass, and myocytic and myofilaments disarray with structurally intact myofibers. The severity of the prognosis is variable and is possibly related to the genotype, depending on the severity of arrhythmias.

The overall strategy followed in the study of this disease is an excellent and representative example of the strategy used for positional cloning. The disease is linked to various mutations located either at different places on the same gene (or locus) (allelic heterogeneity) or on different genes (or locus) in different chromosomes (nonallelic heterogeineity). In other words different genotypes yield the same, or nearly the same, phenotype. The first locus was identified by the group of Christine Seidman

237

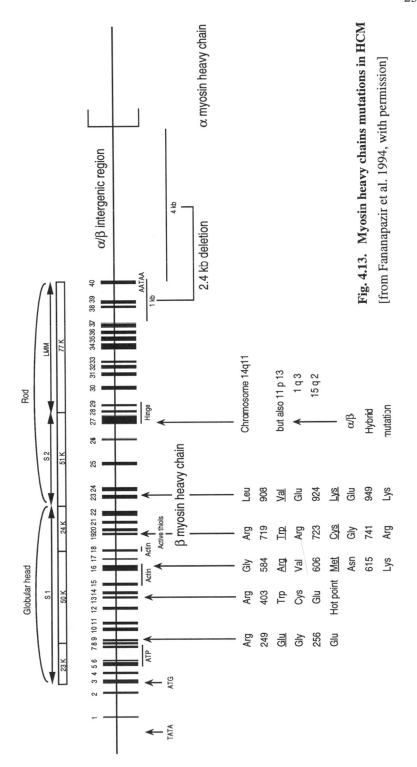

Fig. 4.13. Myosin heavy chains mutations in HCM
[from Fananapazir et al. 1994, with permission]

in 1989 [Jarcho et al. 1989], on chromosome 14 at band q11 by using genetic-linkage analyses. Furthermore, it was demonstrated that, in these kindred, the mutation was a missense $403^{Arg-Glu}$ on exon 13 on the head of the β-isoform of the cardiac myosin heavy chain on the 50 K segment which is close to the actin binding site. Since this pioneer observation, several distinct missense mutations have been reported on the same gene (at least 17 to 20, Figure 4. 12).

More unusual findings included a 2.4 kb deletion representing 10% of the gene, an unequal crossover event occurring during meiosis and resulting in an α/β cardiac myosin hybrid gene (similar hybrids were found in hemoglobinopathy due to hemoglobin P). Other mutations occurring on different loci and different chromosomes [Carrier et al. 1993] include the gene of troponin T (with two missense mutations on exons 8 and 9) on chromosome 1q3, the gene of a-tropomyosin (with a missense mutation in exon 5) on chromosome 15q2, and the gene of protein-C on chromosome 11.

In normal conditions, the β-isomyosin heavy chain gene encodes a protein which is expressed both in the myocardium and in the slow skeletal muscle fibers. In humans, skeletal muscle in general contains a mixture of fast and slow isoforms, and the myosin mutations have also been found in the skeletal muscle [Cuda et al. 1993] in spite of the fact that clinical signs of skeletal myopathy are rare. Purified mutant β-myosin ($908^{Leu-Val}$ and $403^{Arg-Gln}$) isolated from these diseased skeletal muscles had abnormal functions in an *in vitro* assay in which actin filaments are translocated by myosin bound to a coverslip surface.

The relationship with the clinical situation is far from being simple: clinical symptoms such as sudden death or ischemia may result from different mechanisms. Mutations responsible for the disease occur in various part of the genome. The mutation $606^{Val-Met}$, which results in a neutral charge substitution, is malignant in some kindreds whereas it is associated with near normal survival in others. Conversely sudden death occurs in only 2% of the cases with the mutation 256$^{Gly-Glu}$ which results in a charge change. The amino acid 403 is normally an arginine, several different mutations, at least 3, were reported at this particular locus and are associated with a severe prognosis, suggesting that this amino acid is a "hot spot" [Schwartz et al. 1995]. Studies of large kindred is necessary to be certain that a mutation is benign and not accompanied by a high risk of sudden death. To date, only the 908$^{Leu-Val}$ and the 256 $^{Gly-Glu}$ mutations satisfy this requirement .

Because myosin, protein C, tropomyosin, and troponin all lead to the same disease state, one can conclude that FHC can be described best as a disease of sarcomere that an abnormal stoichiometry of sarcomeric protein might be the underlying cause of the hypertrophy, and consequently that FHC is a compensatory hypertrophy. Mutations on myosin, or others components of the contractile apparatus, could poison the assembly of many myosin molecules and result in abnormal contractility. To compensate for such a deficit in contractile state, the heart, as usual, hypertrophies. The skeletal muscle does not hypertrophy because it does not permanently contract, and, in addition, it possesses a fast myosin isoform that may play a compensatory role.

The compensatory hypothesis does not explain the incidence of sudden death nor the asymmetry of the hypertrophy. An intriguing clinical finding is the existence of patients who are proned to sudden death and have cardiac arrhythmias and carry the disease gene but who have no signs of hypertrophy. In other words, the electrical and the morphological forms of the disease can be dissociated. An important issue of the problem is prevention. Could routine genotyping be performed in children or athletes at risk for FHC? The general opinion at present is to reserve routine genotyping to members of a family when a mutation is discovered and not to apply this technique in routine practice. The main reason is our poor knowledge about genotype-phenotype correlations.

Familial dilated cardiomyopathies

Dilated cardiomyopathy is characterised by impaired systolic function and ventricular dilatation. The disease affects 1/2,500 individuals and is a leading indication for cardiac transplantation. Controlled surveys showed a familial form (FDC) in at least 20 to 25% of patients. Genetic analysis of this disease were recent and studies are still incomplete. Different patterns of transmission and variable clinical data suggest that FDC is the final common pathway of a heterogeneous group of disorders [Mestroni 1997].

The most frequent form of FDC is autosomal dominant with low penetrance and characterized by development of ventricular dilatation and dysfunction with progressive failure and severe arrhythmias. Segregation analysis suggest a monogenic disorder, and linkage of the disease was found with chromosome 9 (q13-q22). A second locus was also found on chromosome 1q32. A rare form of FDC is associated with cardiac conduction system disease. Linkage analysis mapped the diseased gene in an Ohio family on chromosome 1 (1p1-1q1) and in a Swiss-German ancestry family on chromosome 3p22-p25. In every case the disease gene is unknown and is under investigation.

The only form of FDC for which the disease gene is known is X-linked FDC (Figure 4. 9). In this condition the disorder is transmitted with the X chromosome (no male-to-male transmission). The mutation has been localized in the promoter region of the dystrophin gene [Milasin et al. 1996]. Dystrophin, a normal component of the cytoskeleton (Figure 2. 15), is reduced in quantity in skeletal muscle, whereas it is undetectable in the myocardium. Other deletions of the same gene have been reported in patients with cardiomyopathy and Becker muscular dystrophy. It is important for the understanding of the pathophysiology of CR that mutations occuring in several other cytoskeleton proteins, including adhalin and vinculin, may cause FDC [reviewed in Mestroni 1997]. Finally, multiple deletions of mitochondrial DNA have also been reported in several families with FDC. There is evidence that there are inherited dilated cardiomyopathy although for the moment no mutations have been identified so far.

Familial arrhythmias

The lengthening of QT interval can be acquired and then is observed in cardiac remodelling as explained above. The long QT syndrome is a rather rare clinically and genetically heterogenous familial disorder that is characterized by a prolongation of the QT interval (QTc interval > 0.44 sec) and a propensity to ventricular arrhythmias and sudden death especially during youth [Moss et al. 1991]. In 1991, 245 different markers were tested and it was shown that two different DNA markers were tightly linked to the disease with a maximum LOD score of 16 at a recombination fraction of zero [Keating et al. 1991]. The Jervell and Lange-Nielsen syndrome is an autosomal recessive disease associated to a bilateral deafness and linked to at least one gene $KvLQV1$ (I_{Ks}). The Romano-Ward syndrome is an autosomal dominant syndrome without deafness that is linked to at least 5 different loci: $KvLQT1$ (I_{Ks}), $HERG$, $SCN5A$ (α-subunit of I_{Na}), $LQT5$ (I_{Ks}), and $LQT4$ which has not been identified.

Arrhythmogenic right ventricular cardiomyopathy is an autosomal dominant disease that is one of the major causes of juvenile sudden death. There are for the moment at least 3 disease loci that have been assigned to chromosome 14q23-q24, 1q42-q43 and 14q12-q22 (close to α-actinin gene).

MULTIGENIC CARDIOVASCULAR DISEASES AND RISK FACTORS

Monogenic diseases are well characterized and delimited topics. Inherited risks factors are of crucial importance in cardiology. Nevertheless, the topic is far from being well defined, and it is, for the moment, only possible to provide several pathways and give examples in a field of investigation where knowledge is increasing day and day. Epidemiological studies have isolated several risk factors, including hyperlipidemias, hypertension, diabetes, and also unknown factors.

Hyperlipidemias

This topic has been recently reviewed in detail [Benlian 1996]. Figure 4. 9. summarizes both the main pathways for lipid transport and metabolism and the main genetic mechanisms responsible for hyperlipidemias.

Lipids are insoluble in the plasma, by definition, and circulate in the blood stream as lipoproteins (LP), which are in a complex of various lipids associated to apoprotein (Apo) [Chan and Boerwinkle 1990]. Dietary lipids are packaged in the intestinal cells and secreted in the lymph as large particles termed *chylomicrons*, using Apo E, Apo C and above all Apo B-100, and are lipolyzed as smaller remnant chylomicrons (exogenous synthesis in figure 4. 10). Endogenous synthesis in the liver results in the formation of very low density LPs, VLDL, and LDL, using apo E, C and above all Apo B-100. LDL are important particles in hyperlipidemias,and mutations in the corresponding apoproteins are major causes of inherited hyperlipidemias. LP(a) is a recently discovered LP that is derived from LDL and includes a specific apo(a) component whose physiological role is unknown but is polymorphic and likely to play an important role in atherogenesis.

LPs deliver lipids to peripheral tissues, and cellular uptake is mediated by receptors that bind the Apo component of LPs. For the moment, several types of LP receptors (Figure 4. 9) have been described (at least four), such as the LP receptors that bind LDL through ApoB and LP receptors specific for ApoE (see above Familial hypercholesterolemia).

There are several classifications for hyperlipidemias. The most popular is that of DS Frederickson, which was proposed in 1967 before the beginning of genetics and which is only based on phenotypic elements [Frederickson et al. 1967] (Table 4. 1).

Table 4. 1. Classification of hyperlipidemias [from Fredrickson et al. 1967; Breslow 1993; Benlian 1996].

Type	Predominant LP	CT	TG	Corresponding familial deficits
I	Chylomicron	+	+++	Apo C-II, LP lipase
IIa	LDL	+++	=	FDA , FH
IIb	LDL + VLDL	++	+	
III	Intermediate DL	++	++	Apo E
IV	VLDL +	++		Apo E
V	Chylomicron ++	+++		Apo E

CT and TG: plasma cholesterol and triglycerides. Apo: apolipoprotein. LP: lipoprotein. LDL and VLDL: low and very low density LP. FDA and FH: familial deficit in apo B-100 and familial hypercholesterolemia.

Genetics of hyperlipidemias includes two different clinical problems. (1) Monogenic hyperlipidemias have been described above, however there are

244

several other rare diseases due to mutations in other apo, such as apo E

Table 4. 2. Genetics of Hyperlipidemias

Low density LP

Apo E phenotype with alleles E4/E3 (population study) ++

Familial defective apo B-100, AD; 3,500$^{Arg\ Glu}$; 1: 500 +

Familial hypercholesterolemia (LDL receptor deficiency), AD; >200 mutations; 1: 500 +

Very low density LP and decreased HDL

Mutation on apo A-I gene (defective HDL)

Defective LP processing: Hepatic lipase, CETP, LP lipase; 1:10^6 (familial chylomicrominemia)

Defective genes controlling HDL catabolism

Apo C-III overexpression (?)

Chylomicrons remnant and intermediary density LP

Dysbetalipoproteinemia (or type III hyperlipidemia), polygenic

ApoE E2/E2 phenotype (1:100), needs environmental factor +

LP (a) level

LP(a) plasma level is genetically determined and may cause hyperlipidemia ++

+ frequent. ++ very frequent. A: autosomal. D: dominant. LP: lipoprotein. Apo: apoLP. 1:500 = frequency in the population. CETP: cholesterol ester transfer protein.

(familial dysbetalipoproteinemia type III), apo A-1, or various lipases or components responsible for the reverse cholesterol transport (Table 4. 2). For example, more than 60 mutations on the unique gene encoding lipoprotein lipase (30 kb, 10 exons) have been reported, including various types of gene rearrangements and point mutations that all cause familial chylomicrominemias type I. (2) Family associations, including complex segregation analysis and path analysis have also demonstrated that 50% of the normal interindividual variability in total cholesterol is associated with polygenic differences [Lusis 1988].

One of the difficulties for appreciating the genetic factor is that the trait - namely, plasma cholesterol or apo content - is highly dependant on environmental factors such as fat or alcohol consumption, exercising, and even smoking habits (which can influence the apo E plasma level). Of particular interest were the family studies that finally evidenced associations between normolipidemic variations and Apo alleles. Three common alleles of apo E designated E2, E3, and E4 have been identified and occur at frequencies of 7, 78 and 15% respectively (Chan et al. 1990). The two most frequently paired alleles are E3/E3 which is shown in 57% of the population, and E4/E3, which is observed in 22% of the population. E2 is associated with lower plasma cholesterol level than E4, and, for example, the mean plasma cholesterol level of the E2/E2 homozygotes is 140 mg/dL, as compared to 197 mg/dL for E4/E4. Such a difference is likely to reflect a faster rate of clearance of the E2 alleles than does the E4 form which is attributable to a diminished clearance of apo E4-bearing lipoproteins by the apo E receptor [Lusis 1988].

Similar studies were performed with apo(a), which is a large glycoprotein associated to apo B-100 in an LDL-like particle termed LP(a). Apo (a) has a structure very similar to that of plasminogen and, both the protein and cDNA contain 15 to 40 copies of a kringle IV-like region, a kringle V-like region, and a variant-protease domain (Figure 4. 10).

There are approximately 40 different isoforms of apo(a) depending of the number of kringles that has been expressed. The length of the protein depends on the number of the kringles and constitutes an inheritable trait. It varies from one individual to another and from one population to another. In addition, the shorter the protein the higher the plasma concentration of LP (a) and the higher the risk of atherosclerosis.

Arterial hypertension

Elevated arterial blood pressure affects 15 to 20% of the adult population. A large variety of genetic and environmental factors contribute to blood pressure elevation, even in single individuals. Studies of monozygotic or dizygotic twins, biologic and adoptive siblings, or larger populations have clearly demonstrated that blood pressure aggregates and suggests an approximate 30% degree heritability for blood pressure. Blood pressure is continuously distributed in the population. The genetic basis of the disease is polygenic, and it is very unlikely that inheritance follows the classical mendelian laws. The trait is quantitative and has been empirically determined as the level of blood pressure (160/95 mmHg), which is accompanied by cardiovascular complications. Taking into account the dimensions of the problem, the genetics of essential arterial hypertension is still a largely unexplored field of investigation.

The candidate gene approach has also been used in the study of hypertension, although on a smaller scale, and the first candidates were the genes coding for the RAS [Soubrier and Cambien 1993]. Linkage, association and sib-pair studies failed to demonstrate any association or linkage between the renin gene and hypertension [Jeunemaître et al. 1992a]. The same negative association or linkage were found for the atrial natriuretic peptide and the Na^+/H^+ antiporter [reviewed in Samani 1994].

By contrast, there is evidence to suggest that such a linkage exists with the angiotensinogen gene: (1) The plasma level of angne is correlated with blood pressure in large epidemiologic studies, especially in young adults. (ii) Linkage studies have been performed using a highly polymorphic and informative (CA) dinucleotide repeat isolated on the angne gene. One of the studies was performed both in Paris and Salt Lake City on 215 pairs of sibs affected by arterial hypertension and another study comes from London and was carried out on 63 mutiplex families. Both demonstrated an excess of concordance for these microsatellite alleles, as compared with the expected concordance if both the disease and the marker segregate independently and conclude that arterial hypertension and the angne are linked and associated [Jeunemaître et al. 1992b; Caulfield et al. 1994]. (3) Several mutations have been detected on the angne gene, and two of them on codons 235 and 174 on exons 2 and 3, gave rise to two pairs of alleles. In one of the above studies [Jeunemaître et al. 1992b] the distribution of the paired alleles was different in hypertensive subjects than in controls and the plasma concentration in angne was correlated with the genotype. Hypertension was not associated with the allelic distribution in the other study [Caulfield et al. 1994].

Significant familial correlations have been found between genetically related individuals and the plasma level of ACE. Once the ACE gene had been cloned, it was shown that this phenotype was associated with an insertion/deletion (I/D) polymorphism located in intron 16 of the gene and that the mean plasma level of DD subjects was about twice that of II subjects. Nevertheless, it was impossible to demonstrate, by sib-pair analysis, any linkage between hypertension and a highly polymorphic marker located close to the ACE gene [Soubrier and Cambien 1993].

Myocardial infarction

One of the most promising features reported in this domain during the last decades was the finding of a linkage between ACE and I/D polymorphism and myocardial infarction [Cambien et al. 1992]. The DD genotype was indeed significantly more frequent in 610 patients with myocardial infarction than in the 733 controls, especially among patients with a low body-mass index and low plasma levels of ApoB (or cholesterol, or cholesterol in LDL) - that is in patients usually considered to be at low risk (with an odd ratio above 3). The DD genotype was not associated with myocardial infarction when risk factors such as smoking habits, plasma levels of ApoA1, LP(a), or fibrinogen were considered. In this particular protocol many patients received drugs affecting blood pressure, and therefore the conclusions of this article do not apply *stricto sensu* to arterial hypertension. This work has a potential interest for drug trial to see if the genotype is related to sensitivity to ACE inhibitors both in terms of blood pressure and survival.

These findings were in contrast to those further reported by Lindpainter [Lindpainter et al. 1995], who showed the same odds ratio to developing coronary disease in physicians with either D/I genotype. Both positive and negative studies continue to accumulate since François Cambien's pioneer work, and there are for the moment no definit answers to the question, except that all studies of patients with diabetes agree on an increased risk of infarction in diabetic patients that carry the ACE DD genotype.

Left ventricular hypertrophy

Epidemiological studies have evidenced left ventricular hypertrophy (LVH) as an independent risk factor linked to cardiovascular and gobal mortality. Genetic studies were so far not conclusive. Schunkert was the first to evidence a link between LVH and the DD genotype, even in patients with normal blood pressure [Schunkert et al. 1994]. Again, both positive and negative (including a negative report from the Framingham cohort) studies accumulate. Interestingly, recent approaches suggest that genetic cofactors could be resposible for these apparent discrepancies.

Diabetes

Type I diabetes is an autoimmune disease caused by several different mutations on different genes encoding the various components of the immune system, including the HLA system at locus HLA-DRB1 on chromosome 6, genes responsible for the maturation and translocation of antigenes, the insulin gene itself, genes coding for the receptors of antigens such as immunoglobulin receptors, or lymphocyte T receptors. There are polymorphic markers linked to the disease and located in the vicinity of the insulin gene. The disease is atherogenic and a major cause of cardiovascular complications [reviewed in Todd 1992 and in Froguel et al. in Corvol et al. 1993].

Type II diabetes is not insulin-dependent. It is an extremely frequent disease (4 to 7% of the population), which is also associated with a high incidence of atherosclerosis, but is not autoimmune. Clinically, this type of diabetes is a major cause of blindness, renal insufficiency, and amputations. The disease is clinically and genetically heterogeneous disorder. Segregation analysis data suggest that type II diabetes is polygenic and results from both the interaction between different gene variants that affect glucose tolerance and environmental factors including obesity and high calorie intake [Froguel et al. 1995]. The genetic approach has been similar to that of arterial hypertension: several rather rare monogenic diseases were first identified, and further the techniques used for multigenic diseases were applied to search new genes or candidate genes.

Maturity onset diabetes of the youth (MODY) is an autosomal dominant heterogeneous type of diabetes due to several different mutations mostly located in the gene encoding glucokinase on chromosome 7p. Until now there are at least 35 different mutations that have been identified on this particular gene. The most frequent mutation is located on exon 7. MODY encompasses several other entities and is also linked to unknown genes located on chromosome 12q (which is associated with a severe form of diabetes) and 20. 1 to 3% of the type II diabetes are due to a single mutation in the mitochondrial DNA for the tRNA^{Leu}. Mitochondrial DNA is located in ovules, and both the disease and the DNA are transmitted by the mother.

The candidate gene approach is actively developed in this area. Good candidates are the genes related to glucose metabolism (at least 40) and mutations have been found in the promotor of insulin, in the insulin receptor (50 mutations were found in the two subunits of the receptor), and in the insulin receptor kinase genes (nevertheless, the link between these two mutations and the disease is rather weak, suggesting that these two genes act as a diabetes suceptibility gene). A single point mutation in the exon 2 of the glucagon gene is associated with type II diabetes and could impair the insulinotropic of glucagon [Froguel et al. 1995].

Nevertheless, the candidate gene aproach has limited applications in such a highly multifactorial disease. A reliable map of thousands of genomic markers is now available and will allow the discovery of new loci linked to type II daibetes.

Obesity

Obesity affects approximately 30% of the population in western countries and represents an independent risk factor for diabetes, hypertension, hyperlipidemia, and coronary artery disease. Morbid obesity appears to have a particularly strong genetic component, and familial obesity is multigenic in nature. The recent demonstration that at least two different genes - namely, leptin [Halaas et al. 1995] and glucagon-like peptide-1 (GLP-1,which is present in the hypothalamus, exendin inhibits the corresponding receptor) [Turton et al. 1996] - reduce feeding which opens an interesting, and rather old, debate about whether obesity results from a genetically determined dysregulation of satiety or of lipolysis and adipose tisue metabolism.

Several possibilities are now currently explored. (1) Efforts have been made to identify the master of adipocyte differentiation to provide a molecular basis for controlling or reversing the development of the disease. The most important transcription factors are an isoform of peroxisome proliferator activated reptors and several CCAAT enhancer binding proteins. Simultaneously several genes responsible for the mouse model of monogenic obesity, including *agouti, ob* and *fat* gene, have been isolated by positional cloning. (2) The β3-adrenergic receptor is located in adipose tissue and plays an important role in the regulation of lipolysis. A Trp64Arg mutation has been identified by the group of D. Strosberg in the corresponding gene in patients having a morbid obesity, and may represent a genetic basis for obesity due to impaired lipolysis [Strosberg 1987]. (3) Leptin is a 16 kD protein that is secreted by adipose tissue in response to an increased caloric uptake. Plasma leptin is indeed increased in the majority of obese patients. Leptin acts as a signal that controls several components that have either orexigen (like neuropeptide Y) or anorexigen properties (like glucocorticoids) and acts as a sort of adipostat. Genetics in this particular area is soon to produce therapeutic developments that are not gene therapy but new concepts concerning the origin of morbid obesity and the regulation of feeding habits.

5

GENE THERAPY AND CELL TRANSPLANT

Gene therapy

Gene therapy is both a promising and fascinating topic as well as a dangerous game by which mankind is trying to more or less substitute for God. For the moment DNA is not a therapy applicable to cardiovascular disease, and it is difficult to predict when such an approach could have a practical output. The domain that is certainly the most promising is that of prevention of restenosis after angioplasty. The purpose of this book is not to extensively review [as in Barr and Leiden 1994; Herrmann 1996; March 1997] a field that is expanding every month, but only to provide the language that permits a full understanding of what is presently on the spot, and to give a few examples.

The list of the clinical gene therapy protocols approved between 1989 and 1995 includes 122 protocols, mostly in phase I, mostly on cancers, with only two protocols on the cardiovascular sytem (on restenosis) [Herrmann 1996]. Strategies currently utilized in such trials include direct action on tumor cells (suicide genes), modification of the innate antitumor activity of the host immune system, and gene transfer to protect normal host tissues from the cytotoxic effects of cancer therapies.

In the future it is most unlikely that gene therapy in cardiology will consist of replacing a diseased gene by a normal sequence, mainly because most of the inherited cardiovascular diseases are multigenic and, for the moment the main targets of this new pharmacology are vessels.The major aim is to try to introduce and then induce the permanent expression of genes able to deliver proteins that would prevent restenosis or thrombosis. Most of the papers recently published are, in fact, attempts to optimize gene transfer in the vessels using reporter genes and various vectors or modes of injection.

Vectors for gene transfer

A explained above retroviruses provide the means of gene transfer, and in the course of evolution viruses have subverted cellular mechanisms to permit entry of viral genes into the cell nucleus. Retroviruses have RNA as their genomic substance (Figure 1. 19) and have been frequently used as vectors to carry the gene of interest (usually termed *expression cassette* - that is a DNA sequence containig the therapeutic gene and an active promotor) (Figure 5. 1). The first step when making a retroviral construct containing an expression cassette is to create the space necessary to introduce the cassette into the viral genome, which necessitates the removal of *gag, pol* and *env* genetic informations. Elimination of this genetic material is done by genetic engineering using a plasmid (step 1, Figure 5. 1). However , deletion of these viral genes means that the virus loses its capacity to assemble into viral particle. Step 2 consists of transfecting the retrovirus DNA vector into a packaging cell line in which the 3 viral genes have been anchored into the genome. The vector, and the expression cassette, are then transcribed into the packaging cell, and a *recombinant* virus is then produced that contains the expression cassette but not the viral genes that contain the genetic informations for the viral structure proteins. Step 3 consists in infecting the target cells which then is able to express the protein of interest, but is unable to produce a new line of virus.

Adenovirus is a DNA virus responsible for either flues or benign ailments. As for retrovirus, the preparation of the DNA construct includes 3 steps and results in a new virus that loses the capacity to multiply. Several groups have tried to transfer genes into the cardiovascular system using such

255

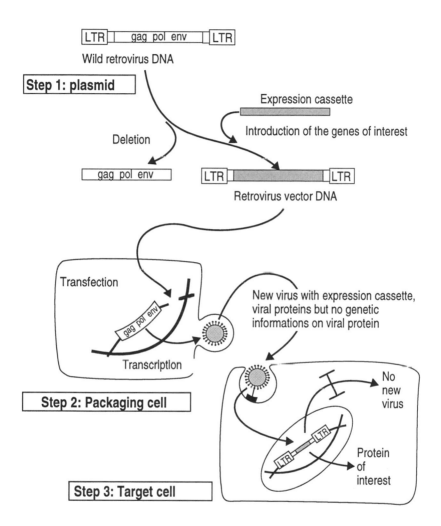

Fig. 5.1. **Retroviral vector system**

a vector. The yield of the transfection is for the moment the highest ever obtained (Barr and leiden 1994; Steg et al. 1994). Nevertheless, the longevity of the transfection seems to be rather limited, and such a vector may create an immune response that has not yet been fully appreciated.

Most of these investigations have been centered around the yield of the transfection using reporter genes. Few of them have, for the moment, used genes of real therapeutic interest. A group of DNA sequences has, however, a particular interest. Antisense sequences or antisense oligonucleotides do indeed have the ability to combine with their complementary (sense) sequences and, consequently, to block gene expression. These sequences have to be combined with a vector to be delivered to the tissue of interest, and, for example, it is now possible to deliver antigrowth factors or antioncogenes oligonucleotides to inhibit the proliferation process responsible for coronary restenosis after PTCA. Antisense c-myb oligonucleotides were, for example, targeted to smooth muscle cells and by so doing inhibit the synthesis of the corresponding oncoprotein with a subsequent effect on the cellular process [Simons et al. 1992]. Obviously, such attempts need parallel progress in the understanding of the biological process responsible for the disease - that is for the latter problem - to understand how the cascade of events responsible for such an anarchic growth is functioning (see Fig. 2. 23). It is, for example, necessary to obtain a greater understanding of the development of the proliferation process after intimal denudation, in the rabbit [Bauters et al. 1994], to more efficiently target arterial gene transfer of DNA sequences.

Liposomal reagents are mixtures of cationic or neutral lipids forming micellar structures in the plasma. They form complexes with DNA and because of their lipidic structure may fuse to the plasma membrane and then deliver the genetic material to the cells. Liposomes are a priori safer than any viral vector since they are entirely artificial structures. Several groups have attempted to transfer reporter proteins into vascular endothelial. This mode of transfection is for the moment poorly efficient [Barr and Leiden 1994; Zhu et al. 1993; March 1997]. One of the surprises of gene therapy is that naked DNA by itself can enter into cells, and skeletal muscle cells appeared a particularly suitable target.

Gene transfer and cell transplant to repair MI

Ventricular remodelling following myocardial infarction refers to the process of early expansion and thinning of the infarcted area that results in progressive dilatation to restore stroke volume and finally cardiac failure. Current therapy to limit infarction size includes early opening of the arteries or using various inhibitors of vasoactive peptides in order to attenuate their excessive vasoactive and trophic effects.

The first experimental approach employs retroviruses as a vector. Retroviruses are able to transduce only in replicating cells and are indeed able to transduce reporter genes in the granulation tissue of the infarcted area, which is rich in proliferative fibroblasts. The following step was to introduce into the diseased area master genes as MyoD, which are able to convert fibroblasts into contractile myotubes. Such a "molecular cardiomyoplasty" [Carpentier et al. 1997] has not for the moment been evaluated in terms of cardiac function.

Another approach consists of engrafting fetal cardiac (using an AT-1 cell line derived from SV40 transformed atrial myocytes) or skeletal myocytes (using cultured myogenic satellite cells) into the infarcted tissue [reviewed in Carpentier et al. 1997]. The first results suggest that this kind of approach may reduce the size of the infarction and improve the functional capacities of the heart [Leor 1997].

CONCLUSION

To write such a book alone was an interesting challenge. I had to summarize both 30 years of research and teaching in the cardiovascular field, and the main tendencies of contemporary research in the domain. In addition, the book was especially addressed to my colleague clinicians, who are usually overloaded with an enormous amount of information, usually written for specialists and not for general practitioners. Thanks to this challenge I learned a lot, particularly in fields such as genetics and genome-based technology, where I was primarily rather ignorant. Nevertheless, the difficulties that I had, for example, in understanding the genetic jargon helped me to try to explain the same jargon to clinicians. I was also obliged to make choices and, for example, to abandon several important sections, such as the energy metabolism or ischemia. It is perhaps rather pretentious to try to draw some lines of conclusion in such a fast-moving field. Nevertheless, I try to summarize my feelings below.

(1) A striking point is the fact that our amount of knowledge's has exploded recently. I personally learned more in this field the last 5 years that during the 25 preceding years. Nevertheless, and curiously, this progress has simplified teaching. Teaching physiology is easier when starting with the molecular anatomy of, for example, the ion channels than by the ion currents and the rather complicated paradigms that are the basis of electrophysiology.

(2) The second point is that, in our domain, the complexity is growing with unbelievable rapidity. To understand how a given patient becomes hyperlipidemic, we should have soon to integrate such an enormous mass of knowledge - including multiallelism (200 alleles for the lipoprotein receptor and 200 genes responsible for the lipid metabolism!) and the environmental biological factors - that it makes us feel dizzy! It is easy to predict that such a complexity will soon require special methods of

analyses capable of integrating the overall data. The future of the modern biology will certainly require the development of more integrative methods.

(3) The third remark concerns new therapeutic approaches. The future of gene therapy will certainly concern more therapy with a gene, such as the prevention of restenosis with antioncogenes, than a substitutive therapy in an inherited disease. In addition, a better understanding of the biological mechanisms responsible for arrhythmias, cardiac failure, or coronary insufficiency will permit a better targeting of the drug design.

(4) Finally, the genome programme will soon oblige the most resistant scientists, as the physiologists, to reconsider their attitude and to evaluate the input of such an incredible amount of new information about their own field of interest, which is an interesting challenge. The knowledge of the genome sequence not only in humans but also in different animal, bacterial, or vegetal species has to the origination of an entirely new approach of biological research. Classical genetics, classical physiology used to proceed from a given physiological function or pharmacological effect on the gene. Investigators now start from the sequence of a key gene for the explored function and look for homologous genes in a sequence databank. Then they try to reconstitute the function.

The RNA display, SAGE, and DNA microarrays methods of analysis allow studies of the ordered and timely expression of nearly all the genes that characterize a given cell and allow differential studies. Such a technological advance provides an unbelievable tool, which now allows the study of the full content of any cell. It is easy to predict that cardiovascular physiology will soon be completely up-and-down by the development of such approaches [Hwang et al. 1997]. Gene classification based on sequence alignments allowed the delineation of protein families based on sequence similarities, and the detection of a particular motif in a sequence data-bank is now a good strategy, especially in pharmacological research, for detecting new functions. The rapid development of cloning procedures, transgenic technology, and transfections leads also to the discovery of a growing amount of new proteins, especially new receptors, whose function becomes progressively known, and again, this has impredictible consequences in terms of biological knowledges.

How to see the forest for the trees in such a jungle? The need for integrative biology is now urgent. A first step consists in developing "functional genomics" as opposed to "structural genomics" [Hieter and Boguski 1997]. *Functional genomics* refers to experimental approaches that assess gene functions by using the information provided by structural genomics. The fundamental new point is that functional genomics aims to study the entire function of a cell by analyzing the overall genetic expression of a given cell or organism. Several new techniques allow indeed a global view of the expression of the entire genome. Powerful examples are the study on yeast, which allows every modification of transcripts (including all the components of the glycolytic pathway and Krebs cycle) to be shown during glucose-depletion [DeRisi et al. 1997] or the entire pattern of genes to be expressed in colon cancer [Zhang et al. 1997]. Another important point is to simplify some extremely complicated schemes (just have a look on the schemes provided on the currently known mammalian MAP kinases pathways, which are, for the moment, the major pathways for cell growth and proliferation) by hierarchizing the component of the pathway and the determinants of cell function. Computer research (bioinformatic) is mandatory for these new approaches, as far are the search and identification of new nonlinear tools that allow the study of the various biological oscillators.

GLOSSARY

adenovirus DNA virus naturally infecting man, frequently used as a vector in gene therapy.

allele One of several alternative forms of a gene that occupies a given locus on the same chromosome. By extension, alternative forms of noncoding (anonymous polymorphism) DNA sequences located on the same locus (Figure 4.1).

anonymous Anonymous DNA is the portion of DNA that does not encode RNAs. It constitutes the majority of DNA sequences, and includes polymorphic markers.

antiparallel See antisense.

antisense An antisense RNA is the mirror copy of a mRNA. In an antisense RNA the nucleotides are arranged in the same order as in the noncoding, antiparallel, DNA strand on which the RNA polymerase synthesizes the mRNA (Figure 1. 9). See also *complementary RNA (cRNA)*.

autosomal Mode of inheritance which is not sex-linked

base pairs (bp) A partnership of nucleotide bases, such as A with T or C with G, in a DNA double strand. A single-stranded sequence of 30 nucleotides is also a double strand of 30 bp.

cell cycle The sequence of events that separates two mitotic or (for gametes) meiotic division in eucaryotes (Figures 1. 3 and 1. 4).

chiasma Chromosomal site where crossing-over occurs (see Figure 1. 4).

chromatin Highly organized structure in which DNA is packaged with proteins (histones). Heterochromatin is permanent dark-staining areas of condensed chromatin in which most of the DNA is never transcribed.

chromosomes Morphologically distinctive nuclear structures, species-specific in number and shape. Assemblies of transcription units made up from DNA,

RNA and proteins, which are precisely duplicated during cell division (Figure 1. 2).

cis/transregulation When transcription is indirectly activated through a protein factor that binds to a DNA responsive element, this is a transregulation; when the activated DNA responsive element enhances transcription, this is a cisregulation (Figures 1. 9 - 1.11).

clone Genetically identical cells descending from a single common ancestral cell

clusters of orthologous groups (COG) COG consist of individual orthologous genes (see ortholog genes) and orthologous sets of paralogs (see paralog genes) which are found in a minimum number of lineages.

coding The genetic code is a special arrangement of bases that allows DNA, which is made from nucleotides, to code for a specific arrangement of amino acids. A given gene or mRNA code for a given protein, but stricto sensu a given DNA sequence, does not code for a given RNA sequence.

codon or triplet a group of three nucleotides that encodes for an amino acid, initiation signal or termination signal (Table 1. 1).

complementary DNA (cDNA) DNA synthesized from a mRNA copy obtained by reverse transcription from mRNAs, tissue-specific by definition. Does not contain introns (Figure 1. 12).

complementary RNA (cRNA) Mirror image of mRNA, also termed antisense RNA and is identical to the antisense DNA strand. Tool made by biotechnology. Exists *in vivo*, but its physiological significance is still unknown (Figure 1. 8). See also *antisense*.

consensus Sequence that is located in the regulatory part of the gene, binds specifically to a given transcriptional factor, and is conserved in various biological species (Figures 1. 9 - 1. 11).

conversion (genetic) Reparation of noncomplementary DNA strand by using the other strand as a guideline (Figure 4. 5).

cross-over Exchange of genetic material between haploid chromosomes that pair during meiosis.

desoxy ribonucleic acid (DNA) Molecule that supports hereditary messages (Figure 1. 5).

diploid A diploid (2n) cell contains two copies of each chromosome. In mammals, as in every eukaryotic organism all, or nearly all the cells, are diploid (Figures 1. 3 - 1. 4).

DNA See desoxy ribonucleic acid

dominant Inheritance is dominant when the expected phenotype is expressed in the heterozygous state.

duplication See replication (Figure 1. 6).

Enhancer Component of the regulatory part of the gene that includes the consensus sequences (Figures 1. 9 - 1. 10).

eukaryote Organism that has nuclei, nuclear membranes, and mitosis.

excision Step of the maturation of mRNAs during which introns are excised. This step is followed by a ligation of the exons (Figure 1. 7).

exon DNA sequence transcribed and found in mature RNA (Figurez 1. 8).

expressed sequence tag (EST) See tag.

5'-3' Indicates the DNA or RNA polarity. A nucleotide consists in a combination of a sugar, a base, and a phosphate group. The bases are attached to the 1' carbon position of the sugar and face the interior of the molecule, while the phosphate group forms the backbone of the molecule and binds to the 5' and 3' carbon position of the sugar. The convention is that the order of the nucleotides is read from 5' to 3', DNA or RNA is synthesized in the 5'-3' direction (Figure 1. 9).

gene All nucleic acid sequences which are necessary to produce a peptide or an RNA. Includes the coding sequences, but also the regulatory sequences (Figures 1. 8 - 1. 10).

genetic code The set of correspondences between codons and amino acids (Table 1. 1).

genetic distance The distance, in centiMorgans, between linked nucleotidic sequences (Figure 4. 3).

genomic DNA Genuine DNA directly extracted from nuclei. It is the same in every cell of a given individual (Figure 1. 12).

genotype The genetic constitution of an individual in terms of DNA sequences (Fig. 1. 1).

germinal cells Gametes (Figure 1. 4).

haploid Haploid cells (1n) contain only one copy of each chromosome (Figures 1. 3 - 1. 4).

hereditary disease A disease caused by a mutant gene (Figure 4. 8).

homology Homologous sequences means sequences sharing many nucleotide sequences in common.

in silico Means through computer analysis.

informative A polymorphic marker is informative when it allows one to identify the father's chromosome from the mother's one and, more particularly, when it allows the localization of a locus on one of these chromosome.

intron A DNA sequence present in premRNA and excluded from mature RNAs. The introns are intercalated between two exons (Figures 1. 7 - 1.8).

kindred Relative.

knock-out Gene transfer technique that consists in blocking the expression of a gene.

lariat After excision the introns appear in the nuclear area as lassos or lariats (Figyre 1. 7).

linkage (genetic) Cosegregation of several alleles due to their physical proximity. Linkage analysis is a method of analysis of inheritance based on the search of a diseased locus using markers (Figures 4. 3, 4. 6).

locus Location, place.

LOD score or log odds ratio Expresses the likehood that two loci are linked at a given recombination frquency. A LOD score above 3 is considered to be significant.

meiosis Germinal cell division (Figure1. 4).

messenger RNA (mRNA) Transcript from which protein can be translated (Figure 1. 7).

mismatch or maipairing Random assignation after crossing-over may give rise to double DNA strands in which one or several bases are not complementary (Figure 4. 5).

missense mutations Mutation in which the codon is mutated to direct the incorporation of a different amino acid.

modules (or domains) Protein building blocks that comprise single or multiple motifs. Example: the ABC transporters consist of two unrelated modules - a pair of ATP-binding cassettes and a pair of membrane-spanning modules. See also *motif*.

motif The smallest sequence unit of protein families. Motifs are identified as highly similar regions in alignments of gene segments. They are used to identify functional regions of proteins. Example: the P-loop motif of the ATP-binding cassette allows the prediction of the presence of ATP binding in a transporter.

mutation Change in a DNA sequence, most often used to qualify a change in the sequence of a gene.

Northern blot A technique used to examine and quantify mRNAs and that is based on electrophoretic separation and hybridization with specific probes (Figure 1. 13). See also *Southern blot*.

nucleosome Basic subunit of chromatin (Figure 1. 2).

offspring Progeny, lineage.

oligonucleotide Synthetic single-stranded nucleotidic sequence (Figure 1. 12).

orphan protein or gene A protein or a gene discovered in a DNA bank and whose function is ignored - for the moment.

ortholog genes Genes in different species that have consostent patterns of sequence similarities, evolve from a common ancestry, and typically perform the same role in different organisms.

palindrome The two DNA strands are complementary and termed palindromic because the two sequences are identical if read from left to right for one strand and right to left for the other. *Ésope reste ici et se repose* is a classical palindromic sentence (Figure 1. 14).

paralog genes Genes related by duplication (of modules, see modules) within a genome.

penetrance The percentage of people having a specif)ied genotype that shows the expected phenotype. Penetrance usually increases with age and is complete when all individuals carrying a given genotype have the expected phenotype.

phage or bacteriophage A virus that infects bacteria. Used as a vector (Figure 1. 18)

phenotype Observable characteristics of an organism resulting from genomic expression. Morphological feature, physiological property, clinical syndrome or protein (Figure 1. 1).

plasmid Extrachromosomal, circular, autonomously replicating DNA segment. Commercially available as a well-defined nucleotidic sequence. Vector.

poly(A) tail Noncoding repetitive sequence of adenine, A, which is synthesized during the maturation of a mRNA, in the nucleus (Figure 1. 7).

polymerase chain reaction (PCR) Qualifies both the technique and the commercially available apparatus used for this technique. The method is an in vitro reproduction of DNA replication (Figure 1. 16).

polymorphism Genomes showing allelic variations. Restriction polymorphism means that the variations modify a restriction site.

primers Single-stranded DNA sequence that is paired with a DNA or RNA strand and provides a free 3' end at which DNA polymerase starts the synthesis of a longer DNA sequence. Exists *in vivo* but is usually synthesized for the purpose of PCR (Figures 1. 6, 1. 16).

probe Biochemical radioactively labeled or tagged for ease of identification (Figure 1. 12).

procaryote Microorganisms that lack a membrane-bound nucleus.

promotor A region of the regulatory part of a gene to which RNA polymerase binds (indirectly) (Figure 1. 9).

protein structure Primary: amino acid sequence; secondary: helical configuration; tertiary: spatial configuration of each chain; quaternary: subunit interaction (Figure 1. 1).

pseudogene Resembles a known functional gene but is rendered nonfunctional by structural changes at crucial points.

recessive Mutation that modifies the phenotype only in homozygotes.

recombinant (1) *In vivo*, at the end of crossing-over recombinants are chromosomes resulting from the reassembly of genes during meiosis (Figure1. 4). (2) In vitro, a recombinant is a composite DNA sequence created by joining foreign DNA with a vector.

recombination frequency Number of recombinants divided by the total number of progeny.

reparation Process by which the cell is able to restaure a normal DNA molecule after injury or recombination, using the other DNA strand as a guideline.

replication DNA synthesis from DNA. The new DNA strands are complementary copies of the DNA templates (Figure 1. 6).

reporter Gene used in a construct to indicate the activity of a promotor of inetrest. The gene usually expresses only proteins that are not normally present in the tissue, such as CAT.

responsive element Consensus nucleotide sequence specific for a given activated transcriptional factor, which is a protein. The element is said to be responsive because it responds to the signal that is transported by the factor. The signal can be hormonal but also mechanical or a signal for differentiation (Figures 1. 10 - 1. 11).

restriction enzymes Endonucleases that cleave unique, specific sequences of duplex DNA. Class II restriction enzymes cleave palindromic sequences (Figure 1. 14).

restriction maps A linear array of sites on DNA cleaved by restriction enzymes. (Figure 1. 15). Commonly utilized to rapidly identify a DNA probe.

retrovirus RNA viruses. These virus are termed *retro*viruses because they use their own reverse transcriptase activity during the cycle when they are transcribed into DNA and integrated into the genome of the host cell. AIDS is caused by a retrovirus HIV. Oncogenic retrovirus are transformants and have the capacity to transform the host cell into a cancerous cell (Figure 1. 19).

ribonucleic acid (RNA) Molecule that is transcribed from DNA.

RNA differential display A PCR method that allows the quantitative analysis of diffentially expressed mRNAs (Figure 1. 21).

rRNA Ribosomal RNA.

SAGE See *serial analysis of gene expression.*

segregate Transmit.

sense Sense RNA is mRNA. Sense DNA strand or noncoding strand is the strand on which the polymerase synthesizes mRNA (Figure 1. 8).

sequencing centers The main centers are the European Molecular Biology Laboratory (EMBL), the National Center for Biotechnology Information (NCBI), the Genome Sequence Data Bank (GSDB), and the DNA Data Bank of Japan (DDBJ).

serial analysis of gene expression (SAGE) This new technique allows the simultaneous quantitation of thousands of transcripts (Figure 1. 22) and is based on two principles: (1) a 9 to 10 bp long nucleotide sequence tag contains sufficient information to uniquely identify a mRNA, provided it is isolated from a define position within the transcript; (2) concatenation of these tags allows the efficient sequencing of these RNAs in a serial manner.

sib-pair analysis Method of analysis of genetic transmission based on paired siblings.

Southern blot The same technique as Northern blot but using DNA fragments instead of RNA. Historically the first, has been described by E.M. Southern in 1975. See Northern blot.

splicing Removal of introns followed by ligation of exons to produce mature translatable mRNAs. Splicing = excision + ligation. Splicing is a mode of regulation of the expression of isoforms (Figure 1. 7).

synapsis A step of meiosis that allows crossing-over.

tag Any short nucleotide sequence, 9 to 10 bp, contains sufficient information to uniquely identify a mRNA, provided it is isolated from a defined position within the transcript. Tags longer than 150 bp were the most usefull for similarity research. Any sequence from a cDNA clone that corresponds to a given mRNA can be called tag. Sequence-tagged sites are standard markers for physical mapping of the human genome and expressed sequence tag (EST) usually qualify the technique which consists in isolating, sequencing, and computer analyzing cDNAs libraries.

taxonomy Science of classification. The pionneer in taxonomy was Linnaeus.

template DNA sequence serving as a model to synthesize RNA or DNA sequence.

trait. Dominant phenotype expression.

transcript mRNA. See *messenger RNA*.

transcription RNA synthesis from DNA.

translation Protein synthesis from mRNA. Translation of a nucleotide sequence into an amino acid sequence. See *messenger RNA*.

transregulation See *cis/trans regulation*.

triplet See *codon* or *triplet*.

upstream A nucleotide sequence is upstream from the coding part of a gene when it is located upstream the initial site of transcription - that is upstream from the 5' end. The regulatory sequences are located upstream from the coding part of the gene.

virus Living elements without nuclei and nuclear membrane and whose genetic material consists of either RNA or DNA.

Western blot Same as Northern or Southern blot but uses antibodies to identify proteins.

yeast artificial chromosomes (YAC) A vector for long sequences

REFERENCES

Adams MD, Kelley JM, Gocayne JD, et al. [1991] Complementary DNA sequencing: expressed sequence tags and human genome project. Science, 252, 1651.

Adler, CP. [1975] Relationship between DNA content and nucleoli in human heart cells and estimation of cell number during cardiac growth and hyperfunction. In Roy PE, Harris P, eds. Recent Advances in Studies on Cardiac Structure and Metabolism. The Cardiac Sarcoplasm. University Park Press, Baltimore, p. 373.

Alpert NR, Mulieri LA. [1982] Increased myothermal economy of isometric force generation in compensated cardiac hypertrophy induced by pulmonary artery constriction in the rabbit. Circ. Res., 491, 50.

Alpert NR, Mulieri LA, Hasenfuss G. [1992] Myocardial chemo-mechanical energy transduction. In Fozzard HA et al., eds. The Heart and Cardiovascular System. Raven press, NwY, p. 111.

Anversa P, Palackal T, Sonnenblick EH, et al. [1990] Myocyte cell loss and myocyte cellular hyperplasia in the hypertrophied aging rat heart. Circ. Res., 67, 871.

APS CV Section. [1997] Beginning the human physiome project. In APS CV Section News. February, p. 3.

Apstein C, Lecarpentier Y, Mercadier JJ et al. [1987] Changes in LV papillary muscle performance and myosin composition with aortic insufficiency in rats. Am. J. Physiol., 253, H1005.

Asano K, Dutcher DL, Port D, et al. [1997] Selective downregulation of the angiotensin II AT1-receptor subtype in failing human ventricular myocardium. Circulation, 95, 113.

Assayag P, Carré F, Chevalier B, et al. [1997a] Compensated cardiac hypertrophy: arrhythmogenecity and the new myocardial phénotype. Part 1: Fibrosis. Cardiovasc. Res., 34, 439.

Assayag P, Charlemagne D, de Leiris J, et al. [1997b] Senescent heart as compared to pressure overload induced hypertrophy. Hypertension, 29, 15.

Barr E, Leiden JM. [1994] Somatic gene therapy for cardiovascular disease. Recent advances. Trends Cardiovasc. Med., 4, 57.

Bauters C, Moalic JM, Bercovici J, et al. [1988] Coronary flow as a determinant of *c-myc* and *c-fos* proto-oncogene expression in an isolated adult rat heart. J. Mol. Cell Cardiol., 20, 97.

Bauters C, Van Belle C, Wernert N et al. [1994] Angiopeptin inhibits oncogen induction in rabbit aorta after ballon denudation. Circulation, 89, 2327.

Becker-André M, Hahlbrock K. [1989] Absolute mRNA quantification using the polymerase chain reaction: a novel approach by a PCR aided Transcription assay (PATTY). Nucleic Acid Res., 17, 9437.

Benlian P. [1993] -6- Dyslipidémies. In Corvol P, Charru A eds., Génétique des maladies cardiovasculaires". Bristol-Myers Squibb cardiovasculaire, Paris, p.71.

Benlian P. [1996] Génétique et dyslipidémies. Approche gène-candidat. Les Éditions INSERM, Paris.

Bertin B, Mansier P, Makeh I, et al. [1993] Specific atrial overexpression of functional human b1-adrenergic receptors in transgenic mice. Cardiovasc. Res., 27, 1606.

Besse S, Assayag P, Delcayre C, et al. [1993] Normal and hypertrophied senescent rat heart. Mechanical and molecular characteristics. Am. J. Physiol., 265, H183.

Besse, S, Delcayre, C, Chevalier B, et al. [1994] Is the senescent heart overloaded and already failing? A review, Cardiovasc. Drugs Ther., 8, 581.

Besse, S, Robert, V, Assayag, P et al. [1994] Non-synchronous changes in myocardial collagen mRNA and protein during aging. Effect of DOCA-salt hypertension, Am. J. Physiol., 267, H2237.

Bing OHL. [1994] Hypothesis: apoptosis may be a mechanism for the transition to heart failure with chronic pressure overload. J. Mol. Cell Cardiol., 26, 943.

Boheler KR, Chassagne C, Martin X, et al. [1992] Cardiac expressions of α- and β-myosin heavy chains and sarcomeric α-actins are regulated through transcriptional mechanisms: Results from nuclear run-on assays in isolated rat cardiac nuclei. J. Biol. Chem., 267, 12979.

Bond RA, Leff P, Johnson TD, et al. [1995] Physiological effects of inverse agonists in transgenic mice with myocardial overexpression of the β2-adrenoceptor. Nature, 374, 272.

Breslow JL. [1993] Genetics of lipoprotein disorders. Circulation, 87 (suppl III), III-16, 1993.

Brilla CG, Pick R, Tan LB, Janicki JS. et al. [1990] Remodeling of the right and left ventricles in experimental hypertension. Circ. Res., 67, 1355.

Bristow MR, Ginsburg R, Minobe W, et al. [1982] Decreased catecholamine sensitivity and beta-adrenergic receptor density in failing human heart. N. Engl. J. Med., 307, 205.

Brodde O-E. [1991] β1- and β2-adrenoceptors in the human heart: properties, function, and alterations in chronic heart failure. Pharmacol. Rev., 43, 203-241.

Brown MS, Goldstein JL. [1986] A receptor-mediated pathway for cholesterol homeostasis. Science, 232, 34.

Brutsaert DL, Sys SU. [1989] Relaxation and diastole of the heart. Physiol. Rev., 69, 1228.

Buttrick PM, Kass A, Kitsis RN et al. [1992] Behavior of genes directly injected into the rat heart *in vivo*. Circ. Res., 70, 193.

Callens-ElAmrani F, Snoeckx L, and Swynghedauw B. [1992] Anoxia-induced changes in ventricular diastolic compliance in two models of hypertension in rats. J. Hypertension, 10, 229.

Cambien F, Poirier O, Lecerf L, et al. [1992] Deletion polymorphism in the gene for angiotensin-converting enzyme is a potent risk factor for myocardial infarction. Nature, 359, 641.

Capasso JM, Malhotra A, Scheuer J, et al. [1986] Myocardial, biochemical, contractile and electrical performance following imposition of hypertension in young and old rats. Circ. Res., 58, 445.

Capecchi MR. [1989] The new mouse genetics: Altering the genome by gene targeting. TIG, 5, 70.

Carpentier A, Chachques JC, Grandjean PA. [1997] Cardiac Bioassist. Bakken Res Center Series. Futura, Armonk, NY.

Carrier L, Hengstenberg C, Beckmann JS, et al. [1993] Mapping of a novel gene for familial hypertrophic cardiomyopathy to chromosome 11. Nature Genetics, 4, 311.

Catterall WA. [1994] Molecular properties of a superfamily of plasma-membrane cation channels. Curr. Op. Cell Biol., 6, 607.

Caulfield M, Lavender P, Farrall M, et al. [1994] Linkage of the angiotensinogen gene to essential hypertension. N. Engl. J. Med., 330, 1629.

Chan L, Boerwinkle E, Li W-H. [1990] Molecular genetics of the plama apolipoproteins. InChien S, ed., Molecular biology of the cardiovascular system. Lea & Fibiger, Philadelphia, p. 183.

Charlemagne D, Maixent JM, Preteseille M, et al. [1986] Ouabain binding sites and (Na+, K+)-ATPase activity in rat cardiac hypertrophy: Expression of the neonatal forms. J. Biol. Chem., 261, 185.

Charlemagne D, Orlowski J, Oliviero P et al. [1994] Alteration of Na, K-ATPase subunit mRNA and protein levels in hypertrophied heart. J. Biol. Chem., 269, 1541.

Chevalier B, Mansier P, Teiger E, et al. [1991] Alterations in β-adrenergic and muscarinic receptors in aged rat heart: Effects of chronic administration of propranolol and atropine. Mech. Aging Dev., 60, 215.

Chidsey CA, Sonnenblick EH, Morrow AG, et al. [1966] Noreprinephrine stores and contractility force of papillary muscle from the failing heart. Circulation, 33, 43.

Chien S., ed. [1990] Molecular Biology of the Cardiovascular System. Lea & Fibiger pub., Philadelphia.

Chomczkynski P, Sacchi N. [1987] Single-step method of RNA isolation by acid guanidium thiocyanate-phenol-chloroforme extraction. Anal. Biochem., 162, 156.

Clapier-Ventura R, Mekhfi H, Oliviero P, et al. [1988] Pressure overload changes cardiac skinned fibers mechanics in rats, not in guinea pigs. Am. J. Physiol., 254, H517.

Collins FS. [1995] Positional cloning moves from perditional to traditional. Nature, 9, 347.

Coraboeuf E. [1978] Ionic basis of electrical activity in cardiac tissues. Am. J. Physiol., 234, H101.

Corman B, Michel JB. [1986] Renin-angiotensin system, converting-enzyme inhibition and kidney function in aging female rats. Am. J. Physiol., 251, R450.

Coronado R, Morrissette J, Sukhareva M, et al. [1994] Structure and function of ryanodine receptors. Am. J. Physiol., 266, C1485.

278

Corvol P, Charru A eds. [1993] Génétique des maladies cardiovasculaires. Bristol-Myers Squibb, Paris.

Coulombe A, Montaza A, Richer P, et al. [1994] Reduction of calcium-independent transient outward current density in DOCA-salt hypertrophied rat ventricular myocytes. Pflügers Arch., 427, 47.

Crie JS, Millward DJ, Bates PC, et al. [1981] Age-related alterations in cardiac protein turnover, J. Mol. Cell. Cardiol., 13, 589.

Cuda G, Fananapazir L, Zhu WS, et al. [1993] Skeletal muscle expression and abnormal function of β-myosin in hypertrophic cardiomyopathy. J. Clin. Invest., 91, 2861.

Cummins P, ed. [1993] Growth Factors and the Cardiovascular System. Kluwer Academic Publishers, Boston.

Danner DB, Holbrook NJ. [1990] Alterations in gene expression with aging. In Schneider EL and Rowe JW eds. Handbook of the Biology of Aging". Academic Press, San Diego, p. 97.

Darnell J, Lodish H, Baltimore D. eds. [1986] Molecular Cell Biology. Scientific American Books, New York.

Davies PF, Tripathi SC. [1993] Mechanical stress mechanisms and the cell. An endothelial paradigm. Circ. Res., 72, 239.

de la Bastie D, Levitsky D, Rappaport L, et al. [1990] Function of the sarcoplasmic reticulum and expression of its Ca $^{2+}$ATPase gene in pressure overload-induced cardiac hypertrophy in the rat. Circ. Res., 554, 66.

de la Bastie D, Moalic JM, Bercovici J, et al. [1987] Messenger RNA content and complexity in normal and overloaded rat heart. Eur. J. Clin. Invest., 17, 194.

Delcayre C, Klug D, Van Thiem N, et al. [1992] Aortic perfusion pressure as early determinant of β-isomyosin expression in perfused hearts. Am. J. Physiol., 263, H1537.

Delcayre C, Samuel JL, Marotte F et al. [1988] Synthesis of stress protein in rat cardiac myocytes 2-4 days after imposition of hemodynamic overload. J. Clin. Invest., 82, 460.

Dell'Italia L, Meng Qc, Balcells E, et al. [1997] Compartmentalization of angiotensin II generation in the dog heart: Evidence for independent mechanisms in intravascular and interstitial spaces. J. Clin. Invest., 100, 253.

DeRisi JL, Iyer VR, Brown PO [1997] Exploring the metabolic and genetic control of gene expression on a genomic scale. Science, 278, 680.

Dinerman JL, Lowenstein CJ, Snyder SH. [1993] Molecular mechanisms of nitric oxide regulation. Circ. Res., 73, 217.

Dubus I, Samuel JL, Marotte F, et al. [1990] β-adrenergic agonists stimulate the synthesis of noncontractile but not contractile proteins in cultured myocytes isolated from adult rat heart. Circ. Res., 66, 867.

Eghbali M, Eghbali M, Robinson TF, et al. [1980] Collagen accumulation in heart ventricles as a function of growth and aging. Cardiovasc. Res., 23, 723.

Erdös T, Butler-Browne GS, Rappaport L. [1991] Mechanogenetic regulation of transcription. Biochimie (Paris), 73, 1219.

Escande D, Standen N, eds. [1993] K+ channels in cardiovascular medicine. Springer-Verlag, Paris.

Eschenhagen, T., Mende, U., Nose, M., et al. [1992] Increased messenger RNA level of the inhibitory G protein a subunit $G_{i\alpha-2}$ in human end-stage heart failure. Circ. Res., 70, 688.

Evans RM. [1988] The steroid and thyroid hormone receptor superfamily. Science, 240, 889.

Fabiato A. [1981] Myoplasmic free calcium concentration reached during the twitch of an intact isolated cardiac cell and during calcium-induced released of calcium from the sarcoplasmic reticulum of a skinned cardiac cell from the adult rat or rabbit ventricle. J. Gen. Physiol., 78, 457.

Fananapazir L, Epstein ND. [1994] Genotype-phenotype correlations in hypertrophic cardiomyopathy. Circulation, 89, 22.

Farhadian F, Contard F, Sabri A, et al. [1996] Fibronectin and basement membrane in cardiovascular organogenesis and disease pathogenesis. Cardiovasc. Res., 32, 433.

Feldman A, Ray PE, Silan CM, et al. [1991] Selective gene expression in failing human heart: Quantification of steady-state levels of messenger RNA in endomyocardial biopsies using the Polymerase Chain Reaction. Circulation, 83, 1866.

Field LJ. [1993] Transgenic mice in cardiovascular research. Annu. Rev. Physiol., 55, 97.

Finch CE, Tanzi RE. [1997] Genetics of aging. Science, 278, 407.

Fleg JL. [1987] Alterations in cardiovascular structure and function with advancing age. Am. J. Cardiol., 57, 33C.

Fleg JL, Kennedy HL. [1982] Cardiac arrhythmias in a healthy elderly population. Chest, 81, 302.

Folkow B, Svanborg A. [1993] Physiology of cardiovacular aging, Physiol. Rev., 73, 725.

Frederickson DS, Levy RI, Lees RS. [1967] Fat transport in lipoproteins - an integrated approach to mechanisms and disorders. N. Engl. J. Med., 276, 34.

Froguel P, Hager J, Vionnet N. [1995] The genetics of type II diabetes. Current Opinion Endocrin. Diabetes, 2, 285.

Ganote C, Armstrong S. [1993] Ischaemia and the myocyte cytoskeleton: review and speculation. Cardiovasc. Res., 27, 1387.

Gauthier C, Tavernier G, Charpentier F, et al. [1996] Functional β3-receptor in the human heart.J. Clin. Invest., 98, 556.

Gidh-Jain M, Huang B, Jain P, et al. [1996] Differential expression of voltage-gated K^+ channel genes in left ventricular remodeled myocardium after experimental myocardial infarction. Circ. Res., 79, 669.

Gilman AG. [1987] G proteins: transducers of receptor generated signals. Annu. Rev.Biochem., 56, 615.

Gomez AM, Valvidia HH, Cheng H, et al. [1997] Defective excitation-contraction coupling in experimental cardiac hypertrophy and heart failure. Science, 276, 800.

Grépin C, Durocher D, Nemer M. [1995] Le coeur: un programme unique de transcription et de différenciation musculaire. Médecine/Sciences (Paris), 11, 395.

Gros DB, Jongsma HJ. [1996] Connexins in mammalian heart function. BioAssays, 18, 719.

Gwathmey JK, Copelas L, MacKinnon R, et al. [1987] Abnormal intracellular calcium handling in myocardium from patients with end-stage heart failure. Circ. Res., 61, 70.

Gwathmey JK, Slowsky MT, Haijar RJ et al. [1990] Role of the intracellular calcium handling in force-interval relationships of human ventricular myocardium. J. Clin. Invest., 85, 1599.

Hanf R, Drubaix I, Lelièvre L. [1988] Rat cardiac hypertrophy: altered sodium-calcium exchange activity in sarcolemmal vesicles. FEBS Letters, 236, 145.

Hansen PS, Rüdiger N, Tybjaerg-Hansen A et al. [1991] Detection of the apo B-3500 mutation (glutamine for arginine) by gene amplification and cleavage with MspI. J. Lipid Res., 32, 1229.

Hardouin S, Bourgeois F, Besse S, et al. [1993] Decreased accumulation of β1-adrenergic receptors, $G_{\alpha S}$ and total myosin heavy chain messenger RNAs in the left ventricle of senescent rat heart. Mech. Aging Develop., 71, 169.

Hart, G. [1994] Cellular electrophysiology in cardiac hypertrophy and failure. Cardiovasc. Res., 28, 933.

Harvey RP, Olson EN, Schulz RA, Altman JS, eds. [1997] Genetic Control of Heart Development. HFSP, Strasbourg.

Hasenfuss G, Holubarsch, C, Just H, Alpert NR eds. [1992] Cellular and Molecular Alterations in the Failing Human Heart. Steinkopff Verlag, Darmstadt.

Hathaway DR, March KL, Lash JA, et al. [1991] Vascular smooth muscle. A review of the molecular basis of contractility. Circulation, 83, 382.

Hatt PY, Berjal G, Moravec J, et al. [1970] Heart failure: an electron microscopic study of the left ventricular papillary muscle in aortic insufficiency in the rabbit. J. Mol. Cell Cardiol., 1, 235.

Hatt PY, Ledoux C, Bonvalet JP. [1965] Lyse et synthèse des protéines myocardiques au cours de l'insuffisance cardiaque expérimentale. Arch. Mal. Coeur Vx., 12, 1703.

Hefti MA, Harder BA, Eppenberger HM, et al. [1997] Signaling pathways in cardiac myocyte hypertrophy. J. Mol. Cell Cardiol., 299, 2873.

Heistad DD, Fakunding J. [1997] Special emphasis panel on integrative research. Circulation, 95, 1977.

Henikoff S, Greene JEA, Pietrokovski S, et al. [1997] Gene families: the taxonomy of protein paralogs and chimeras. Science, 278, 609.

Herrmann F. von Harsdorf R, Lang RE, Fullerton M et al. [1989] Myocardial stretch stimulates phosphatidyl inositol turnover. Circ. Res., 65, 494.

Heyliger CE, Prakash AR, McNeill JH. [1988] Alterations in membrane Na^+-Ca^{2+} exchange in the aging myocardium. Age, 11, 1, 1.

Heymes C, Silvestre JS, Llorens-Cortes C, et al. [1998] Cardiac senescence is associated is associated with enhanced expression of angiotensin II receptor subtypes. Endocrinology, 139, 2579.

Heymes C, Swynghedauw B, Chevalier B. [1994] Activation of angiotensinogen and angiotensin converting enzyme gene expression in the left ventricle of senescent rats. Circulation, 90, 1328.

Hieter P, Boguski M. [1997] Functional genomics: it's all how you read it. Science, 278, 601.

Hirzel H, Tuchsmid C, Sneider J et al. [1985] Relationship between myosin isoenzyme composition, hemodynamics and myocardial structure in various forms of human cardiac hypertrophy. Circ. Res., 57, 729.

Holtzman NA, Murphy PD, Watson MS, et al. [1997] Predictive genetic testing: from basic research to clinical practice. Science, 278, 602.

Hwang DM, Dempscy AA, Wang R-X, et al. [1997] A genome-based resource for molecular cardiovascular medicine. Toward a compendium of cardiovascular genes. Circulation, 96, 4146.

Isoyama S, Wei JY, Izumo S. et al. [1987] Effect of age on the development of cardiac hypertrophy produced by aortic constriction in the rat. Circ. Res., 61, 337.

Iwase M, Bishop SP, Uechi M, et al. Heymes C, Silvestre JS, Llorens-Cortes C, et al. [1996] Adverse effects of chronic endogenous sympathic drive induced by cardiac $G_{\alpha s}$ overexpression. Circ. Res., 78, 517.

Izumo S, Nadal-Ginard B and Mahdavi V. [1988] Proto-oncogene induction and reprogramming of cardiac gene expression produced by pressure overload. Proc. Natl. Acad. Sci. USA, 85, 339.

Jarcho JA, McKenna W, Pare P et al. [1989] Mapping a gene for familial hypertrophic cardiomyopathy to chromosome 14_q1. N. Engl. J. Med., 321, 1372.

Jeunemaître X, Rigat B, Charru A, et al. [1992a] Sib-pair linkage analysis of renin gene haplotypes in human essential hypertension. Hum. Genet., 88, 301.

Jeunemaître X, Soubrier F, Kotelevtsev YV et al. [1992b] Molecular basis of human hypertension: Role of angiotensinogen. Cell, 71, 169.

Kajstura J, Cheng W, Reiss K, et al. [1996] Apoptotic and necrotic myocyte cell deaths are independent contributing variables of infarct size in rats. Lab. Invest., 74, 86.

Kaplan J-C, Delpech M, eds. [1993] Biologie Moléculaire et Médecine. Médecine-Sciences/Flammarion, Paris.

Katusic ZS and Shepherd JT. [1991] Endothelium-derived vasoactive factors: II Endothelium-dependent contraction. Hypertension, 18 (Suppl III), III-86.

Keating M, Atkinson D, Dunn C et al. [1991] Linkage of a cardiac arrhythmias, the long QT syndrome, and the *Harvey ras-1* gene. Science, 252, 704.

Kelly RA, Balligand J-L, Smith TW. [1996] Nitric oxide and cardiac function. Circ. Res., 79, 363.

Koch WJ, Rockman HA, Samama P, et al. [1995] Cardiac function in mice overexpressing the β-adrenergic receptor kinase or β-ARK inhibitor. Science, 268, 1350.

Kretsinger RH, Barry CD. [1975] The predicted structure of the calcium-binding component of troponin. Biochem. Biophys. Acta, 405, 40.

Kriegler M ed. [1990] Gene Transfer and Expression. A Laboratory Manual. M. Stockton Press, New York.

Kurihara Y, Kurihara H, Suzuki H et al. [1994] Elevated blood pressure and craniofacial abnormalities in mice deficient in endothelin-1. Nature, 368, 703.

Lakatta, E. [1993] Cardiovascular regulatory mechanisms in advanced age. Physiol. Rev., 73, 413.

Lalli E, Sassone-Corsi P. [1994] Signal transduction and gene regulation: the nuclear response to cAMP. J. Biol. Chem., 269, 17359.

Lauer B, Thiem NV, Swynghedauw B. [1989] ATPase activity of the cross-linked complex between cardiac myosin subfragment 1 and actin in several models of chronic overloading. Circ. Res., 64, 1106.

Leclercq JF, Swynghedauw B. [1976] Myofibrillar ATPase, DNA and hydroxyproline content of human hypertropied heart. Eur. J. Clin. Invest., 6, 27.

Lelièvre L, Maixent JM, Lorente P, et al. [1986] Prolonged responsiveness to ouabaïn in hypertrophied rat heart: Physiological and biological evidence. Am. J. Physiol., 250, H923.

Leor J, Prentice H, Sartorelli V, et al. [1997] Gene transfer an cell transplant: an experimental approach to repair "broken heart". Cardiovasc. Res., 35, 431.

Liang P, Pardee AB. [1992] Differential display of eucaryotic messenger RNA by means of the polymerase chain reaction. Science, 257, 967.

Lifton RP. [1996] Molecular genetics of human blood pressure variations. Science, 272, 676.

Lindpainter K, Pfeffer MA, Kreutz R, et al. [1995] A prospective evaluation of an angiotensin converting enzyme gene polymorphism and the risk of ischemic heart disease. N. Engl. J. Med., 332, 706.

Lingrel JB, Kuntzweiler T. [1994] Na^+, K^+-ATPase. J. Biol. Chem., 269, 19659.

Lompré AM, Lambert F, Lakatta EG., et al. [1991] Expression of sarcoplasmic reticulum Ca^{2+}ATPase and calsequestrine genes in rat heart during ontogenic development and aging, Circ. Res., 69, 1380.

Lompré AM, Nadal-Ginard B, Mahdavi V. [1984] Expression of the cardiac ventricular α and β myosin heavy-chain genes is developmentally and hormonally regulated. J. Biol. Chem., 255, 6437.

Lompré AM, Schwartz K, d'Albis A et al. [1979] Myosin isozymes redistribution in chronic heart overloading. Nature, 282, 105.

Lotersztajn S. [1993] Les endothélines. Médecine/Science (Paris), 9, 1084.

Lüscher TF, Boulanger CM, Dohi Y, et al. [1992] Endothelium-derived contracting factors. Hypertension, 19, 117.

Lusis AJ. [1988] Genetic factors affecting blood lipoproteins: the candidate gene approach. J. Lipid Res., 29, 397.

Mangin L, Swynghedauw B, Benis A et al. [1998] Relatiosnhips between heart rate and heart rate variability. Study in conscious rats. J. Cardiovasc. Pharmacol., in press.

MansierP, Chevalier B, Barnett DB, et al. [1993] Beta adrenergic and muscarinic receptors in compensatory cardiac hypertrophy of the adult rat. Pflügers Arch., 424, 354.

Mansier P, Médigue C, Charlotte N, et al. [1996] Decreased heart rate variability in transgenic mice overexpressing atrial ß1-adrenoceptors. Am. J. Physiol., 271, H1465.

Maquart FX, Gillery P, Klais B, et al. [1994] Cytokines and fibrosis. Eur. J. Dermatol., 4, 91.

March KL, ed. [1997] Gene Transfer in the Cardiovascular System. Experimental Approaches and Therapeutic Implications. Kluwer Academic Publishers, Boston.

Marie JP, Guillemot H, Hatt PY. [1976] Le degré de granulation des cardiocytes auriculaires. Etude planimétrique au cours des différents apports d'eau et de sodium chez le rat. Pathol. Biol. (Paris), 24, 549.

Marks AR, Taubman MB ed. Molecular biology of cardiovascular disease. Marcel Dekker pub. NwY. 1997.

Meerson FZ. [1969] The myocardium in hyperfunction hypertrophy. Circ. Res., 25 (suppl. II).

Meerson FZ, Javich MP, Lerman MI. [1978] Decrease in the rate of RNA and protein synthesis and degradation in the myocardium under long term compensatory hyperfunction and on aging. J. Mol. Cell. Cardiol., 10, 145.

Mercadier JJ, de la Bastie D, Ménasché P, et al. [1987] Alpha-myosin heavy chain isoform and atrial size in patients with various types of mitral valve dysfunction: a quantitative study. J. Am. Coll. Cardiol., 9, 1024.

Mercadier JJ, Samuel JL, Michel JB et al. [1989] Atrial natriuretic factor gene expression in rat ventricle during experimental hypertension. Am. J. Physiol., 257, H979.

Mestroni L. [1997] Dilated cardiomyopathy: a genetic approach. Heart, 77, 185.

Michel J-B, Mercadier JJ, Galen FX, et al. [1990] Urinary cyclic guanosine monophosphate as an indicator of experimental congestive heart failure in rats. Cardiovasc. Res., 24, 946.

Milano CA, AllenLF, Rockman HA, et al. [1994] Enhanced myocardial function in transgenic mice overexpressing the β2-adrenergic receptor. Science, 264, 582.

Milasin J, Muntoni F, SeverinI GM, et al. [1996] A point mutation in the 5' splicing site of the dystrophin gene first intron responsible for X-linked dilated cardiomyopathy. Hum. Mol. Genet., 5, 73.

Moalic JM, Bercovici J, Swynghedauw B. [1984] Heavy chain and actin fractional rats of synthesis in normal and overloaded rat heart ventricles. J. Mol. Cell Cardiol., 16, 875.

Moalic JM, Charlemagne D, Mansier P, et al. [1993] Cardiac hypertrophy and failure, a disease of adaptation. Modifications in membrane proteins provide a molecular basis for arrhythmogenicity. Circulation, 87 (suppl IV), IV21.

Mondry A, Bourgeois F, Carré F, et al. [1995] Decrease in β1-adrenergic and M2-muscarinic receptor mRNA levels and unchanged accumulation of mRNAs coding for $G_{\alpha i-2}$ and $G_{\alpha s}$ proteins in rat cardiac hypertrophy. J. Mol. Cell Cardiol., 27, 2287.

Morad M, Ebashi S, Trautwein W, Kurachi Y, eds. [1996] Molecular physiology and pharmacology of cardiac ion channels and transporters. Kluwer Academic Publishers Boston.

Moss AJ, Schwartz PJ, Crampton RS et al. [1991] The long QT syndrome. Prospective longitudinal study of 328 families. Circulation, 84, 1136.

Nabel EG, Plantz G, Boyce FM et al. [1989] Recombinant gene expression *in vivo* within endothelial cells of the arterial wall. Science, 244, 1342.

Nio, Y., Matsubara, H., Murasawa, S., et al. [1995] Regulation of gene transcription of angiotensin II receptors subtypes in myocardial infarction. J. Clin. Invest., 95, 46.

O'Brien PJ, Gwathmey JK. [1995] Myocardial Ca^{2+}- and ATP-cycling imbalances in end-stage dilated and ischemic cardiomyopathies. Cardiovasc. Res., 30, 394.

Orchard CH, Lakatta EG. [1985] Intracellular calcium transients and developed tension in rat heart muscle. J. Gen. Physiol., 86, 637.

Pashmforoush M, Chien KR. [1997] Tangled up in blue. Molecular cardiology in the postmolecular era. Circulation, 96, 4126.

Peng CK, Buldyrev SV, Goldberger AL, et al. [1992] Long-range correlation in nucleotide sequences. Nature, 356, 168.

Pepin MC, Pothier F, Barden N. [1992] Impaired type II glucocorticoid-receptor function in mice bearing antisense RNA transgene. Nature, 355, 725.

Peters TJ, Wells G, Oakley CM, et al. [1977] Enzymic analysis of endo-myocardial biopsy specimens from patients with cardiomyopathies. Br. Heart J., 39, 1333.

Pieske B, Kretschmann B, Meyer M, et al. [1995] Alterations in intracellular calcium handling associated with the inverse force-frequency relation in human dilated cardiomyopathy. Circulation, 92, 1169.

Pool PE, Chandler BM, Sonnenblick EH, et al. [1968] Integrity of energy stores in cat papillary muscle. Circ. Res., 22, 213.

Quaini F, Cigola E, Lagrasta C, et al. [1994] End-stage cardiac failure in humans is coupled with the induction of proliferating cell nuclear antigen and nuclear mitotic division in ventricular myocytes. Circ. Res., 75, 1050.

Rakusan K, Nagaï J. [1994] Morphometry of arterioles and capillaries in hearts of senescent mice. Cardiovasc. Res., 28, 969.

Rappaport L, Samuel JL. [1988] Microtubules in cardiac myocytes. Int. Rev. Cytol., 113, 101.

Regitz-Zagrosek V, Friedel N, Heymann A, et al. [1995] Regulation, chamber localization, and subtype distribution of angiotensin II receptors in human hearts. Circulation, 91, 1461.

Reithmeier RAF. [1994] Mammalian exchangers and co-transporters. Current Opinion Cell Biol., 6, 583.

Robert R, ed. [1993] Molecular Basis of Cardiology. Blackwell Scientific, Cambridge, Ma, 1993.

Robert V, Besse S, Sabri A, et al. [1997] Differential regulation of Matrix Metalloproteinases associated with aging and hypertension in the rat heart. Lab. Invest., 76, 729.

Robert V, Thiem NV, Cheav SL, et al. [1994] Increased cardiac types I and III collagen mRNAs in aldosterone-salt hypertension. Hypertension, 24, 30.

Roden DM, George AL Jr. [1997] Structure and function of cardiac sodium and potassium channels. Am. J. Physiol., 273, H511.

Rowen L, Mahairas G, Hood L. [1997] Sequencing the human genome. Science, 278, 605.

Sainte-Beuve C, Allen PD, Dambrin G, et al. [1997] Cardiac calcium release channel (ryanodine receptor) in control and cardiomyopathic human hearts: mRNA and protein contents are differentially regulated. J. Mol. Cell Cardiol., 29, 1237.

Samani NJ. [1994] Molecular gentics of susceptibility to the development of hypertension. Br. Med. Bul., 50, 260.

Sambrook J, Fritsch EF, Maniatis T. [1989] Molecular cloning: A laboratory manual. Cold Spring Harbor Laboratory Press, Cold Spring Harbor, NJ.

Samuel JL, Barrieux A, Dufour C et al. [1991] Reexpression of a foetal pattern of fibronectin mRNAs during the development of rat cardiac hypertrophy induced by pressure overload. J. Clin. Invest., 88, 1737.

Scamps F, Mayoux E, Charlemagne D et al. [1990] Ca current in single isolated cells from normal and hypertrophied rat heart. Effect of b adrenergic stimulation. Circ. Res., 67, 199.

Schaper J, Speiser B. [1992] The extracellular matrix in the failing human heart. In Hasenfuss G, Holubarsch, C, Just H, and Alpert NR, eds. Cellular and Molecular Alterations in the Failing Human Heart, Steinkopff Verlag, Darmstadt, p. 303.

Schena M, Shalon D, Heller R, et al. [1996] Parallel genome analysis: microarray-based expression monitoring of 1000 genes. Proc. Natl. Acad. Sci. USA, 93, 10614.

Schiaffino S, Samuel JL, Sassoon D, et al. [1989] Non-synchronous accumulation of α-skeletal actin and β myosin heavy chain mRNAs during early stages of pressure overload-induced cardiac hypertrophy demonstrated by in situ hybridization. Circ. Res., 64, 937.

Schott RJ, Morrow LA. [1993] Growth factors and angiogenesis. Cardiovasc. Res., 27, 1155.

Schunkert H, Hense HW, Holmer SR, et al. [1994] Association between a deletion polymorphism of the angiotensin converting enzyme gene and left ventricular hypertrophy. N. Engl. J. Med., 330, 1634.

Schwartz JB, Gibb WJ, Tran T. [1991] Aging effects on heart rate variation. J. Gerontol., 46, M99.

Schwartz K, Carrier L, Guicheney P, et al. [1995] Molecular basis of familial cardiomyopathies. Circulation, 91, 532.

Schwartz K, Lecarpentier Y, Martin JL, et al. [1981] Myosin isoenzymic distribution correlates with speed of myocardial contraction. J. Mol. Cell. Cardiol., 13, 1071.

Shepherd JT, Katusic ZS. [1991] Endothelium-derived vasoactive factors: I Endothelium-dependent relaxation. Hypertension, 18 (Suppl III), III-76.

Shiojima I, Yamazaki T, Komuro I, et al. [1996] Molecular aspects of mechanical stress-induced cardiac hypertrophy and failure. In Sasayama S ed., New Horizons for Failing Heart Syndrome. Springer, Tokyo, p. 3.

Silvestre JS, Robert V, Heymes C, et al. [1998] Myocardial production of aldosterone and corticosterone in the rat. J. Biol. Chem. 273, 4883.

Simons M, Edelman ER, DeKeyser JL et al. [1992] Antisense c-myb oligonucleotides inhibit intimal arterial smooth muscle cell accumulation in vivo. Nature, 359, 67.

Simpson PC, Karns LR, Long CS. An approach to the molecular regulation of cardiac myocyte hypertrophy. In Chien S ed., Molecular Biology of the Cardiovascular System, Lea & Fibiger, Philadelphia.

Sing CF, Moll PP. [1990] Genetics of atherosclerosis. Annu. Rev. Genet., 24, 171.

Snoeckx LHEH, Contard F, Samuel JL, et al. [1991] Expression and cellular distribution of heat-shock and nuclear oncogene proteins in rat heart. Am. J. Physiol., 261, H1443.

Sohal RS, Weindruch R. [1997] Oxidative stress, caloric restriction, and aging. Science, 273, 59.

Soubrier F, Alhenc-Gelas F, Hubert C et al. [1988] Two putative active centers in human angiotensin I-converting enzyme revealed by molecular cloning. Proc. Natl. Acad. Sci. 85, 9386.

Soubrier F, Cambien F. [1993] Renin-Angiotensin system genes as candidate genes in cardiovascular diseases. Trends Endocrinol. Metabol., 3, 250.

Spooner PM, Brown AM, eds. [1994] Ion channels in the cardiovascular system. Function and dysfunction. Futura, Armonk, NY.

Steg PG, Feldman, LJ, Scoazec JY et al. [1994] Arterial gene transfer to rabbit endothelial and smooth muscle cells using percutaneous delivery of an adenoviral vector. Circulation, 90, 1648.

Stratford-Perricaudet LD, Makeh I, Perricaudet M et al. [1992] Widespread long-term gene transfer to mouse skeletal muscle and heart. J. Clin. Invest. 90, 626.

Strosberg AD. [1987] Molecular and functional properties of beta-adrenergic receptors. Am. J. Cardiol., 59, 3F.

Studer R, Reinecke H, Bilger J et al. [1994] Gene expression of the cardiac Na^+-Ca^{2+} exchanger in end-stage human heart failure. Circ. Res., 75, 443.

Sütsch G, Brunner UT, von Schulthess C, et al. [1992] Hemodynamic performance and myosin light chain-1 expression of the hypertrophied left ventricle in aortic valve disease before and after valve replacement. Circ. Res., 70, 1035.

Swynghedauw B. [1986] Developmental and functional adaptation of contractile proteins in cardiac and skeletal muscle. Physiol. Rev., 66, 710.

Swynghedauw B ed. [1990] Cardiac hypertrophy and failure. INSERM-J. Libbey, Paris-London.

Swynghedauw B ed. Biologie Moléculaire. Principes et Méthodes. Nathan. Paris, 1994b.

Swynghedauw B Transgenic models of myocardial dysfunction. Heart Failure Rev., 1, 277, 1996.

Swynghedauw B, Barrieux A. [1993a] An introduction to the jargon of molecular cardiology. Part I. Cardiovasc. Res., 27, 1414.

Swynghedauw B, Chevalier B, Charlemagne D et al. [1997] Cardiac hypertrophy, arrhythmogenicity, and the new myocardial phenotype. II. The cellular adaptational process. Cardiovasc. Res., 35, 6.

Swynghedauw B, Coraboeuf E. [1994a] Basic aspects of myocardial function, growth, and development. Cardiac hypertrophy and failure. In Willerson JT and Cohn JN. eds., Cardiovascular Medicine. Churchill Livingstone, New York, p. 771.

Swynghedauw B, Moalic J-M, Bourgeois F, et al. [1993b] An introduction to the jargon of molecular biology. Part II. Cardiovasc. Res., 27, 1566.

Taegtmeyer H, Overturf ML. [1988] Effects of moderate hypertension on cardiac function and metabolism in the rabbit. Hypertension, 11, 416.

Tatusov RL, Koonin EV, DJ Lipman [1997] A genomic perspective on protein families. Science, 278, 631.

Tedgui A, Levy B eds. [1994] Biologie de la paroi artérielle, Paris.

Todd JA. [1992] Diabetes mellitus. Curr. Opin. Genet. Develop., 2, 474.

Tsutsui H, Ishihara K, Cooper G IV. [1993] Cytoskeletal role in the contractile dysfunction of hypertrophied myocardium. Science, 260, 682.

Tybjaerg-Hansen A, Humphries SE. [1992] Familial defective apolipoprotein B100: a single mutation that causes hypercholesterolemia and premature coronary artery disease. Atherosclerosis, 96, 91.

Urata H, Boehm KD, Philip A, et al. [1993] Cellular localization and regional distribution of an angiotensin II-forming chymase in the heart. J. Clin. Invest., 91, 1269.

294

van Bilsen M, Chien KR. [1993] Growth and hypertrophy of the heart: towards an understanding of cardiac specific and inducible gene expression. Cardiovasc. Res., 27, 1141.

Velculescu VE, Zhang L, Vogelstein B et al. [1995] Serial analysis of gene expression. Science, 270, 484.

von Harsdorf R, Lang RE, Fullerton M et al. [1989] Myocardial stretch stimulates phosphatidyl inositol turnover. Circ. Res., 65, 494.

von Harsdorf R, Schott RJ, Shen YT et al. [1993] Gene injection into canine myocardium as a useful model for studying gene expression in the heart of large mammals. Circ. Res., 72, 688.

Wang A, Doyle MV and Mark DF. [1989] Quantification of mRNA by the polymerase chain reaction. Proc. Natl. Acad. Sci., 86, 9717.

Wang X, Feuerstein GZ. [1997] The use of mRNA differential display for discovery of novel therapeutic targets in cardiovascular disease. Cardiovasc. Res., 35, 414.

Watson JD, Hopkins NH, Roberts JW, et al eds. [1987] Molecular Biology of the Gene. Benjamin/Cummings, Menlo Park, CA.

Weber KT, Brilla CG. [1991] Pathological hypertrophy and cardiac interstitium: Fibrosis and renin-angiotensin-aldosterone system. Circulation, 83, 1849.

Weber KT, Brilla CG, Janicki JS. [1993] Myocardial fibrosis: its functional significance and regulatory factors. Cardiovasc. Res., 27, 341.

Weissenbach J. [1996] Le grand tournant des programmes génomes. C.R. Acad. Sci. Paris, 319, 247.

Williamson JR, Monck JR. Second messengers of inositol lipid metabolism and calcium signaling. In Fozzard HA et al eds., The heart and Cardiovascular System. Raven Press, New York, p. 1729.

Wingender E ed. [1993] Gene Regulation in Eukaryotes. VCH, New York.

Wolff JA, Malone RW, Williams P et al. [1990] Direct gene transfer into mouse muscle *in vivo*. Science, 247, 1465.

Yamazaki T, Komuro I, Nagai R et al. [1996] Stretching, the evidence in the case of cardiac growth. Cardiovasc. Res., 31, 493.

Yanagisawa M, Kurihara H, Kimura S, et al. [1988] A novel potent vasoconstrictor peptide produced by vascular endothelial cells. Nature, 332, 411.

Zeiher AM. [1996] Endothelial vasodilator dysfunction: Pathogenic link to myocardial ischemia or epiphenomenon. Lancet 348 (suppl I), s10.

Zhang L, Zhou W, Velculescu VE, et al. [1997] Gene expression profiles in normal and cancer cells. Science, 276, 1268.

Zhu N, Liggit D, Liu Y et al. [1993] Systemic gene expression after intravenous DNA delivery into adult mice. Science, 261, 209.

INDEX